Mother and Child Care

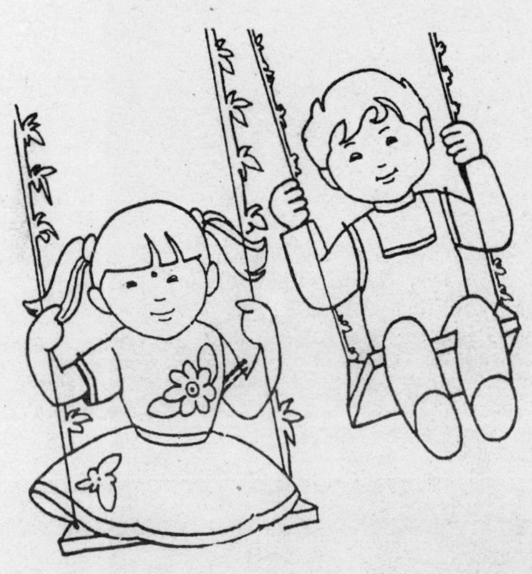

A successful consultant is one who borrows your watch to tell you the correct time. A religious guru is one who sits by the side of a river and sells bottled river water at a premium.

Mother and Child Care

DR. L. C. GUPTA M.D., D. Sc (Hon)
DR. SUJATA M.S., M. CH., D.N.B
DR. KUSUM GUPTA M.A., L.L.B., Ph. D. (Hon)

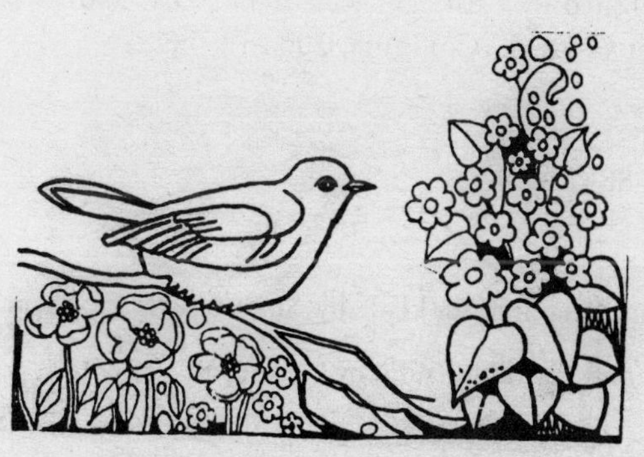

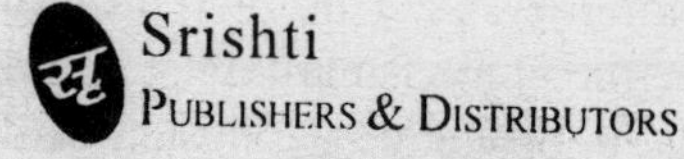
Srishti
PUBLISHERS & DISTRIBUTORS

Srishti Publishers & Distributors
64-A, Adhchini
Sri Aurobindo Marg
New Delhi 110 017
srishtipublishers@yahoo.com

First published by Srishti Publishers & Distributors in 2004

ISBN 81-88575-27-5

Typeset in AGaramond 11pt. by Suresh Kumar Sharma at Srishti

Printed and bound in India by

Cover design by Sandip Sinha
Email: sundeepsinha@yahoo.co.in

Dedicated

to

My First Love

"KUSUM"

AND

"ROHAN"

(For whom

'Ba' means Baba

&

'Baba' means 'Bazar')

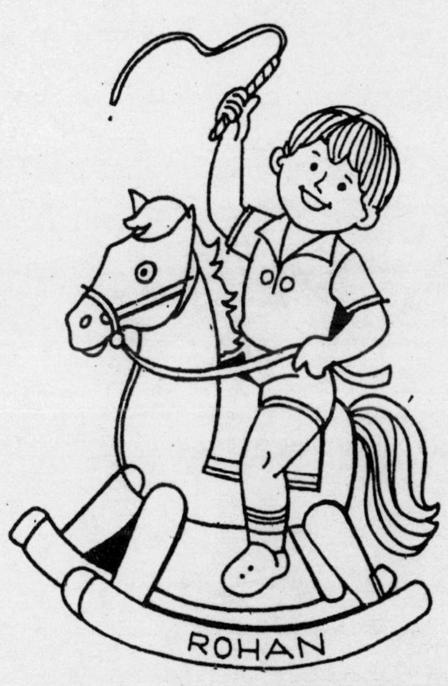

> Hugs, smiles and laughter are more effective parenting tools and will mean more to your child in the long run than most marvellous toys or chocolates.

Contents

Section – I

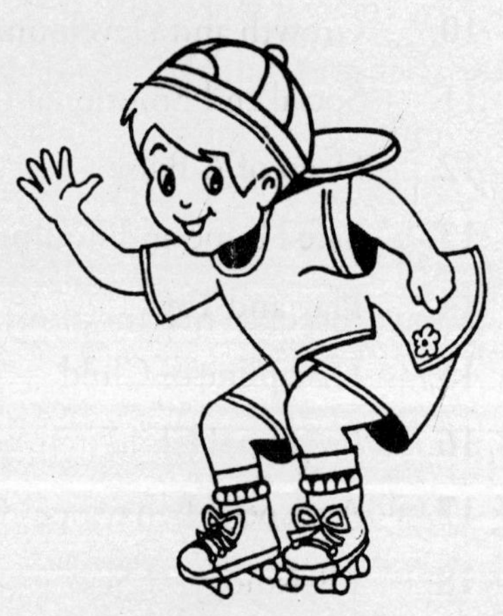

Preface

World Health Organizations (WHO) has played a dynamic role in creating and inculcating awareness about health and better health-condition of humankind. It has also played a helpful role in establishing infrastructure, disease control and better management in developing as well as developed countries. However, it can not be denied that much remains to be achieved for the weaker sections of the communities in these countries. Lack of adequate resources is a handicap but people's cooperation can help achieve some of the objectives and targets. Population control, child care and mother's health care are some features which can lead to overall improvement in health.

Today it is accepted that child care is a harmonious blend of science and art and adequate parental care does develop an infant into a good human being. Understanding child psychology is the first step for the growth of the child and securing his potential – a real reward for the parents and the society. (We have used a 'he' for the child in this book for matter of convinience. This does not reflect any bias.)

We have attempted in this book to cover the various aspects of child care – a child's emotional and psychological needs, physical growth at different stages, age groups, immunisation, diseases and treatment.

Some of our friends – Dr Jad Aoun of Lebnan, Mrs Mani Raj Sharma, Dr Ila Gupta, Dr Archana Dayal, Dr S. K. Acharya, Dr Vandana Mangal and reputed acupressurist Dr A. K. Saxena –

helped us with their suggestions and expert advice which we gratefully acknowledge. We also thank the artists who have contributed to this volume and Ravindra Gupta of Need Book Depot.

Book has been compiled under the aegis of Shankuntala Devi Multi Therapy Health and Research Foundation.

L. C. Gupta
Sujata
Kusum

Good father brings out the best in child.

Section One

Becoming A Mother

Dr. L. C. Gupta

What is spermatozoa?

It is 1/25th of a millimetre long. It consists of a head, a neck and a tail.

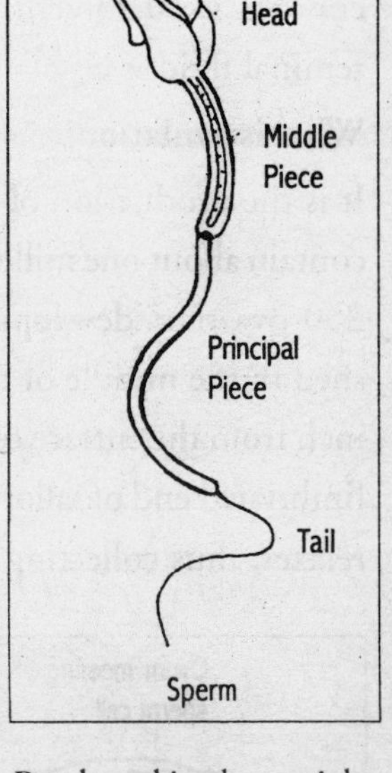

The head measures 1/25th of a millimetre in diametre and contains the chromosomes that fertilize the ovum. Its neck is cylindrical and short and helps in movements. The tail is 10-15 times longer than head The tail is thin, narrow and tapering. It propels the sperm with a side to side movement.

Where sperms are stored?

Spermatogenesis is the formation of sperm. Life of a sperm is 2-3 months.

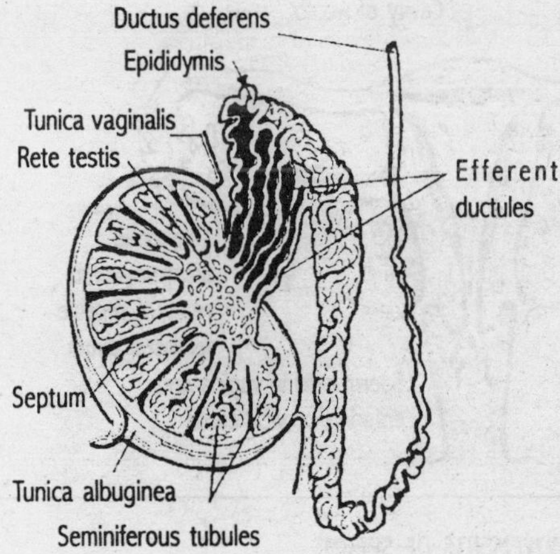

TESTIS

Produced in the testicles it reaches the epididymis where it remains for several days. From the epididymis sperms reach via vas-deference, seminal vesicles. It lies at the base of the bladder where sperms are stored until ejaculation. Prostate secretion with seminal vesicles make the seminal fluid.

What makes ejaculation?

Ejaculation occurs at the time of male orgasm. It consists of muscular contractions. Seminal vesicles contract and emit the seminal fluid containing sperm into male urethra. Ejaculation consists 4-10 forceful contractions. During each contraction seminal fluid is ejaculated from the penis.

What is ovulation?

It is the production of an egg by an ovary. Ovaries of newborns contain about one million ova. During each menstrual cycle about 250 ova start developing. Out of these only one ripens and is shed in the middle of the cycle. When ova is ripe it bulges ½ an inch from the surface of ovary. On ruptuse ovum reaches into the fimbriated end of fallopian tube. The muscular wall contracts and relaxes; thus collecting and guiding the fluid and ovum into the

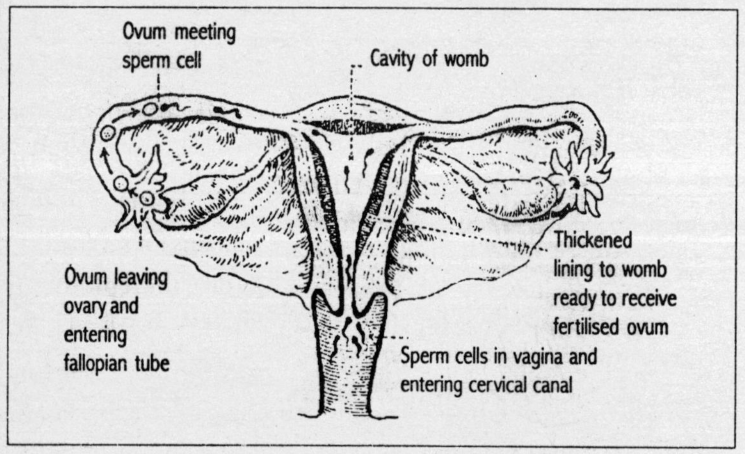

MOVEMENTS OF SPERMS

tube where fertilisation takes place. Life of an unfertilised ovum lasts about 12 to 18 hours. If not impregnated, it gets fragmented and is absorbed by the fallopian tube.

Ovulation occurs generally on 14th day of a 28 day menstrual cycle.

How sperms travel?

Approximately 200-400 million sperms are present in each ejaculation. Semen is semigelatinous which liquifies within 15-20 minutes. Acidity of cervical canal either kills or makes the sperms immobile. For a few days cervical fluid especially becomes transparent and less viscous.

How many sperms reach the cervix?

Only 10% sperms reach the cervical canal after completing their journey of 23 centimetres up to the fallopian tubes. About 1000-2000 sperms reach the outer portion of the fallopian tubes. The tubes secrete an alkaline mucus rich in sugar which nourishes the sperms during their journey of 48 to 72 hours in the fallopian tubes.

What is the need of so many sperms?

Ovum is surrounded by a gelatinous material. This can be liquefied by hyaluronidase which is an enzyme carried by the sperms. A single sperm does not carry enough of hyaluronidase to liquefy the gelatinous material to penetrate the ovum. In order to penetrate the ovum the hyaluronidase of several sperms is needed.

What is the mechanism of penetration of ovum by a sperm?

Exact mechanism is not known till today but a sperm makes direct head-on contact with the ovum. It penetrates the wall due to its hard swimming velocity. A tail of sperm does not enter the ovum.

What do you understand by implantation?

On 7th day chorionic villi develops. Chorionic villi burrow into

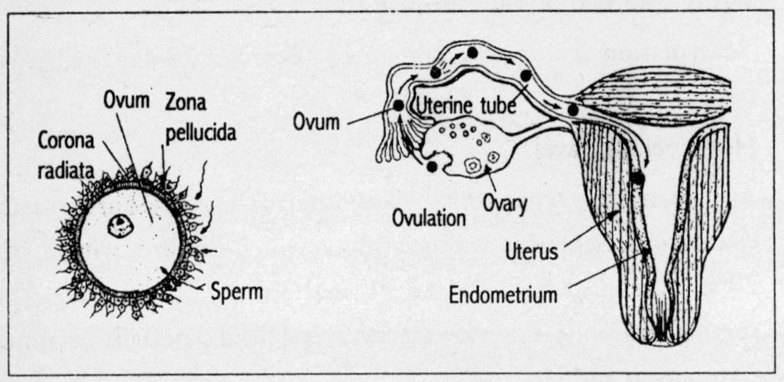

superficial cells of the uterus which they digest and erode. Implantation of fertilised ovum is usually in the upper and posterior part of uterus.

What factor decides the sex of the child?

Human cell contains 46 chromosomes. Of these two are sex chromosomes. The other 44 chromosomes are responsible for hereditary characteristics.

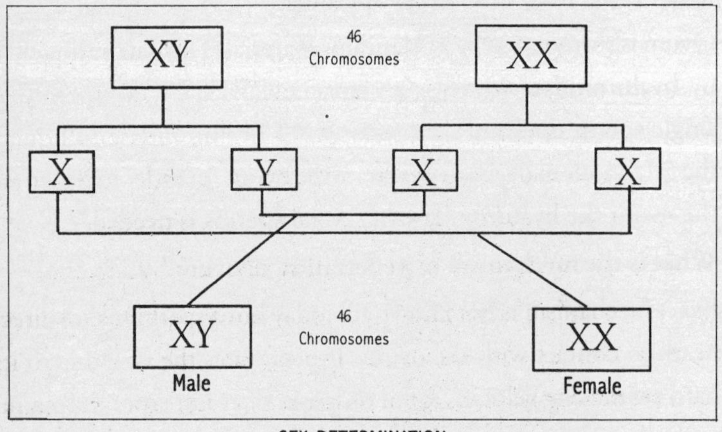

SEX DETERMINATION

A female cell contains two 'XX' chromosomes while a male cell contains 'XY'.

The ovum contains 22 chromosomes plus one sex 'X' chromosome. Each sperm contains 22 chromosomes plus one either 'X' or 'Y' sex chromosome. If the ovum is fertilised by a sperm which contains 22 plus one X chromosome, the fertilised ovum will have 44 plus two XX chromosomes. In this case the child would be female. On the other hand if the ovum is fertilised by a sperm containing one 'Y' sex chromosome the offspring will be male.

Does predestination play role in formation of sex?

No, there is no evidence that the production of male and female children are hereditary phenomenon. Satistically each pregnancy stands an equal chance of being male or female.

Are male and female resulting sperms different?

Yes, their characteristics are different. Female sperms are less motile

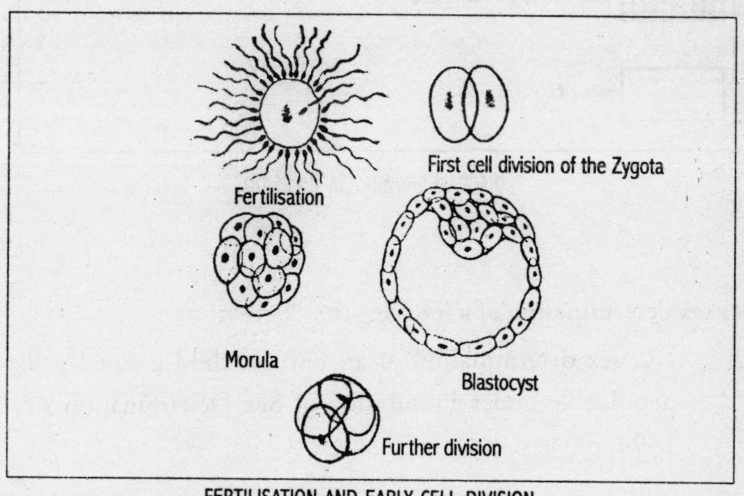

FERTILISATION AND EARLY CELL DIVISION

and they survive for a longer period. If intercourse takes place on day 12 then only female sperms will survive to fertilise the egg on the 14th day. If coitus takes place on the 14th day then chances are that male sperms will reach faster to fertilise. The ovum survives for 12 to 18 hours.

What is the safe period?

A safe period is that phase of a menstrual cycle when conception is least likely to result from intercourse even without the use of contraceptive devices.

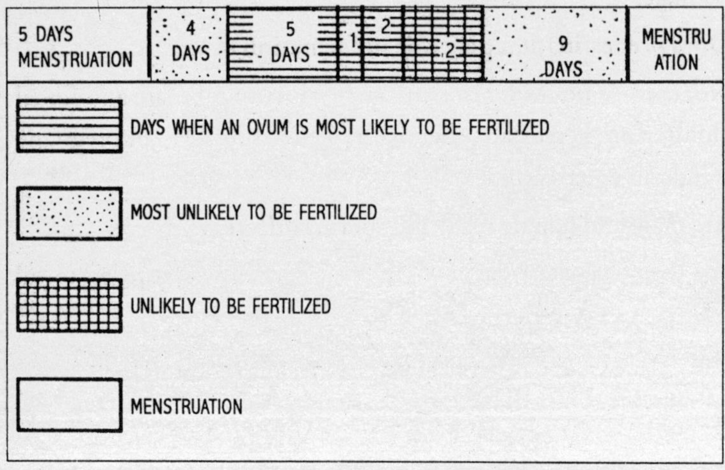

DIAGRAM SHOWING SAFE PERIOD

Is sex determination of a fetus legal?

- No, sex determination of an unborn child is not legally permissible under Prohibition of Sex Determination Act 1994.

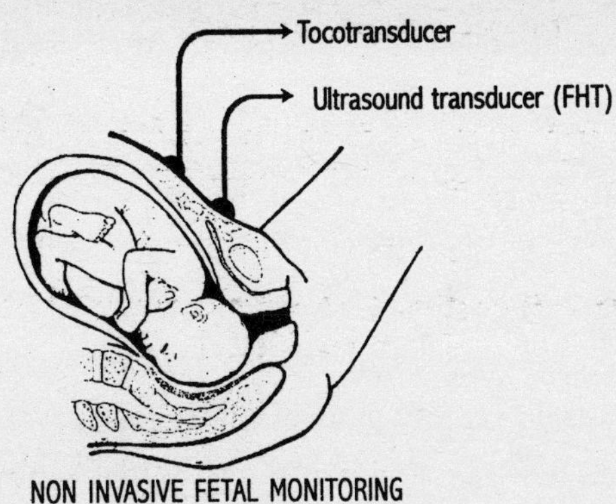

NON INVASIVE FETAL MONITORING

- Utilisation of ultrasonography, amniocentasis to determine the sex of an unborn child is punishable under the Law of January 1996. Doctors indulging in these tests can be imprisoned for five years and fined up to Rs. 1,0C,000.
- Use of Pre Natal Dignostic Techniques are allowed only for detecting abnormalities, disorders and congenital anomaly.

Modern love is being able to walk arm in arm, even when you don't see eye to eye.

Early Symptoms of Pregnancy

Dr. Sujata

What do you understand by amenorrohoea?

Not to have menstruation is the first sign of pregnancy during child bearing age while having regular intercourse. Missed menstrual period is commonly presumed to be due to pregnancy.

What are the other probable causes of cessation of menstrual cycle?

In addition to pregnancy tuberculosis, diabetes, severe anemia, stress, strain and sudden shocking news may result in missed menstrual period.

What do you understand by partially suppressed periods?

If production of progesterone is little, small amount of uterine bleeding may occur in early pregnancy. Such periods are scanty and of shorter duration without any pain. Under such circumstances diagnosis becomes difficult.

Do women feel nausea?

Sensation of feeling sick is very common specially during the first three months of pregnancy. In some women it is the first sign of pregnancy. Each woman has her own pattern of feeling nausea. Some may suffer most of the day. Exact cause of nausea is not known. Nausea decreases after the 10th week of pregnancy. Diet control and anti histamines will help.

What do you understand by 'morning sickness'?

Severe vomiting in the early morning may be troublesome specially when the stomach is empty. Excessive vomiting is known as hyperemesis gravidorum and may require treatment in hospital. Vomiting itself does no harm to the mother or the child. Have some sweet tea or a piece of sweet early in the morning which can help the mother. Fats should be avoided.

What is the position of micturition during pregnancy?

There will be an increase in frequency of micturition. She may be passing urine 4-6 times. There will be no pain and discomfort. Frequency of micturition may be reduced during 4th month but it may again increase after the 7th month.

Do some woman develop constipation during pregnancy?

Constipation is not a sign of pregnancy. But progesterone may relax the intestinal muscles producing constipation in some women.

What type of change in taste develops during pregnancy?

There is a strange taste in mouth. Some describe it as a metallic taste. While some develop dislike of cigarettes or tobacco, some cannot tolerate the smell of cooking fat.

What skin changes takes place during pregnancy?

Some women develop spots on their faces. These spots go away and the complexion returns to normal soon but in some cases it may persist for a longer period. The nipple enlarges and becomes more prominent. There is dilatation of veins over breasts.

What do you understand by quickening?

Quickening is the feeling of fetal movements which is a good sign of pregnancy. Movements are better felt during 16-18th week.

What changes takes place in the uterus in pregnancy?

Uterus measures about 7 centimetre in length, 5 centimetre in width and over 2.5 centimetre in thickness. The weight of the uterus increases throughout pregnancy. It increases from 40 grams to 800 grams, about 40 times.

What changes takes place in the vagina?

Blood supply to the vagina increases. Certain amount of congestion also occurs. Vaginal secretions begin to increase early in pregnancy resulting in mucoid discharge. If there is an infection this secretion may become profuse and offensive. There may be soreness and irritation.

Does blood pressure rise during pregnancy?

Slowing in the circulation causes a fall in blood pressure during early pregnancy. This may lead to light headedness.

After about 14 weeks the blood pressure returns to normal. Any abnormal rise of blood pressure is the first sign of pre eclampsia.

What is a phantom pregnancy?

It is a false pregnancy where the women will complaint of all the symptoms of pregnancy. It generally occurs in some women who have lost a child or a pregnancy. It may be an emotional reaction.

Antenatal Care

Dr. Archana Dayal

- Aim of antenatal care in pregnancy is to maintain good health of the mother during pregnancy. It is concerned with health education during pregnancy.

What is the aim of the first visit to an antenatal clinic?

The aim is to register yourself with the doctor and his team who will look after you during your pregnancy. Details may be inquired about your family history of twin pregnancy, diabetes, hypertension or any type or form of congenital deformity.

Doctors will record information about your previous pregnancies. Your body weight, blood pressure will be checked and a blood examination for hemoglobin will be done.

What is the role of height, weight, urine test?

A woman with the height of less than 5 feet may not have an adequate pelvis. Regular gain in body weight during different months is to be noted. During the whole pregnancy about 11 to 12 kilogram of body weight is gained. You may be advised a diet to maintain proper weight. Mid stream sample of urine may be taken to rule out diabetes and protein (albumin) in urine.

Why per vaginal examination is done during pregnancy?

- To confirm the presence of pregnancy.
- To confirm the size of uterus.
- To ensure that pregnancy is normal.
- To exclude any infection of vagina/cervix.
- To assess the size of cavity of pelvis.
- To exclude any other abnormality.

What blood tests are done during antenatal clinic?

Certain blood tests are vital

(i) Hemoglobin estimation is the density of red blood cells in blood. It is denoted in grams as a percentage. Normal level is 13 gram percentage but may go down to 10-11 gram percentage. If it falls below this level, then the person is said to be anemic.

(ii) A test for checking the blood grouping A, B, AB or O will be done to know the group of the person in advance because if there is a need for blood transfusion then this will be useful.

(iii) It is important to know if the woman is Rhesus negative or positive. If negative, a test may be done for Rhesus antibodies.

(iv) Wassermann reaction is done to test for syphilis. Syphilis is a disease which can be transmitted to the unborn child after 20th week of pregnancy.

Do pregnant ladies require more of iron and vitamins?

Prescribing iron and folic acid after 3 months of pregnancy is common in India, specially folic acid which prevents a particular type of anemia occuring in pregnancy.

Why subsequent visits are necessary to antenatal clinics?

Visits are usually planned every four weeks until the 28th week of pregnancy. At each visit you will be weighed, your urine will be tested, your blood pressure taken and recorded.

Ultrasound will be done on the 16th week. This will help in confirming the duration of pregnancy.

As pregnancy progresses the normal progress of milestones are carefully recorded. After the 28th week the doctor can feel the baby lying in the uterus and can define its exact position.

Does fundal height gives indication of duration of pregnancy?

Yes, at 12 weeks the uterus can be palpated 1-2 centimetre above

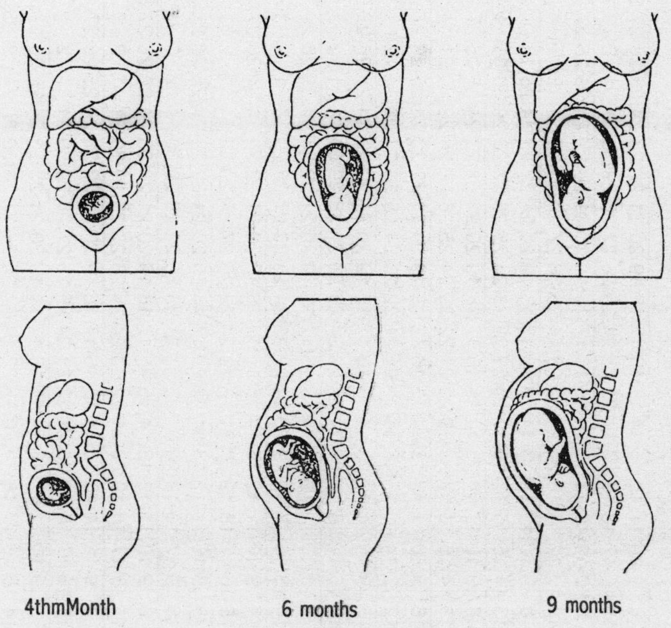

FETUS AT DIFFERENT AGE OF GESTATION

symphysis. At 16 weeks the uterus can be palpated between symphysis and umbilicus. At 24 weeks it is located 1-2 finger above umbilicus. At 36 week the uterus can be located 1 finger below xiphoid process.

Estimating Your Baby's Date of Birth

January	1	2	3	4	5	6	7	8	9	10	11	12	13	14	15	16	17	18	19	20	21	22	23	24	25	26	27	28	29	30	31	Jaunary
October	8	9	10	11	12	13	14	15	16	17	18	19	20	21	22	23	24	25	26	27	28	29	30	31	1	2	3	4	5	6	7	November
February	1	2	3	4	5	6	7	8	9	10	11	12	13	14	15	16	17	18	19	20	21	22	23	24	25	26	27	28				February
November	8	9	10	11	12	13	14	15	16	17	18	19	20	21	22	23	24	25	26	27	28	29	30	1	2	3	4	5				December
March	1	2	3	4	5	6	7	8	9	10	11	12	13	14	15	16	17	18	19	20	21	22	23	24	25	26	27	28	29	30	31	March
December	6	7	8	9	10	11	12	13	14	15	16	17	18	19	20	21	22	23	24	25	26	27	28	29	30	31	1	2	3	4	5	January
April	1	2	3	4	5	6	7	8	9	10	11	12	13	14	15	16	17	18	19	20	21	22	23	24	25	26	27	28	29	30		April
January	6	7	8	9	10	11	12	13	14	15	16	17	18	19	20	21	22	23	24	25	26	27	28	29	30	31	1	2	3	4		February
May	1	2	3	4	5	6	7	8	9	10	11	12	13	14	15	16	17	18	19	20	21	22	23	24	25	26	27	28	29	30	31	May
February	5	6	7	8	9	10	11	12	13	14	15	16	17	18	19	20	21	22	23	24	25	26	27	28	1	2	3	4	5	6	7	March
June	1	2	3	4	5	6	7	8	9	10	11	12	13	14	15	16	17	18	19	20	21	22	23	24	25	26	27	28	29	30		June
March	8	9	10	11	12	13	14	15	16	17	18	19	20	21	22	23	24	25	26	27	28	29	30	31	1	2	3	4	5	6		April
July	1	2	3	4	5	6	7	8	9	10	11	12	13	14	15	16	17	18	19	20	21	22	23	24	25	26	27	28	29	30	31	July
April	7	8	9	10	11	12	13	14	15	16	17	18	19	20	21	22	23	24	25	26	27	28	29	30	1	2	3	4	5	6	7	May
August	1	2	3	4	5	6	7	8	9	10	11	12	13	14	15	16	17	18	19	20	21	22	23	24	25	26	27	28	29	30	31	August
May	8	9	10	11	12	13	14	15	16	17	18	19	20	21	22	23	24	25	26	27	28	29	30	31	1	2	3	4	5	6	7	May
Septermber	1	2	3	4	5	6	7	8	9	10	11	12	13	14	15	16	17	18	19	20	21	22	23	24	25	26	27	28	29	30		September
June	8	9	10	11	12	13	14	15	16	17	18	19	20	21	22	23	24	25	26	27	28	29	30	1	2	3	4	5	6	7		July
October	1	2	3	4	5	6	7	8	9	10	11	12	13	14	15	16	17	18	19	20	21	22	23	24	25	26	27	28	29	30	31	October
July	8	9	10	11	12	13	14	15	16	17	18	19	20	21	22	23	24	25	26	27	28	29	30	31	1	2	3	4	5	6	7	August
November	1	2	3	4	5	6	7	8	9	10	11	12	13	14	15	16	17	18	19	20	21	22	23	24	25	26	27	28	29	30		November
August	8	9	10	11	12	13	14	15	16	17	18	19	20	21	22	23	24	25	26	27	28	29	30	31	1	2	3	4	5	6		September
December	1	2	3	4	5	6	7	8	9	10	11	12	13	14	15	16	17	18	19	20	21	22	23	24	25	26	27	28	29	30	31	December
Septermber	7	8	9	10	11	12	13	14	15	16	17	18	19	20	21	22	23	24	25	26	27	28	29	30	1	2	3	4	5	6	7	October

How to determine expected date of delivery?

Add seven days to the date of the last menstrual period. Substract three months. This gives the date of delivery.

Ready made charts are also available.

How much rest does the mother need when she is pregnant?

It varies with so many personal factors. Best is rest for 8 hours in bed at night and 2 hours in bed in afternoon. During early pregnancy one feels unduely tired. After the 14th week one start feeling better, i.e. less tired and more energetic. Then again during the last 3 months one feels the need for more rest.

What about the pattern of sleep?

Tiredness is one of the natural phenomenon of pregnancy. After one month one feels lassitude. As pregnancy advances sleep usually becomes lighter. The mother wakes more easily. Fetal movements may disturb her when she is asleep. The irritable bladder may wake her during night. Conjestion in nose may be more annoying and cultivation of mental and physical relaxation is necessary. Sleeping pills should be avoided.

What about dreams during pregnancy?

During pregnancy one dreams more. This may be caused by lighter sleep. Disturbed sleep and increased micturition during pregnancy may contribute to an increased frequency of dreams.

What is the role of walking during pregnancy?

There is no limit to walking during pregnancy. But one should not go on hiking expeditions. While walking always stop when you feel tired.

Can one swim during pregnancy?

With certain precautions one can swim. Swimming in very cold water is not advisable because it may cause cramps. Diving from a height is also not advisable.

Can a pregnant lady take part in dancing?

Light dance can be continued with sufficient precautions. Aerobic dancing is to be avoided. Dancing may be reduced as pregnancy advances.

Is cycling permitted during pregnancy?

Cycle riding can be done at any stage of pregnancy. Although during early pregnancy reflexes slow down. As pregnancy advances woman's blance can be affected due to enlarged abdomen.

Is fresh air needed during pregnancy?

Amount of oxygen and other constituents are identical inside and outside a well ventilated house. The psychological effect of getting out is beneficial. Short walks bring freshness.

Is lifting of weight advisable during pregnancy?

Lifting of heavy weights is not advisable. One can lift light weights in which extra effort is not needed. One should not bend to lift objects. It is better to lift by squatting down. Lifting a child can be tiring and risky.

Is travelling allowed in pregnancy?

One may not travel over a long distance or otherwise when the journey is likely to be jerky. Travelling by comfortable train is permitted and preferred over travelling going in a car for more than a 100 miles. Driving a motor cycle is not safe.

Travelling should be avoided if pregnancy is not stable or if the mother is bleeding, or if she has suffered from a miscarriage in the past.

During the last 6 weeks even travel by air is not advisable.

Can one take travel pills?

Majority of pills are manufactured to control travel sickness and are very similar to the ones which are given to control morning sickness. If you travel during the time period of morning sickness it may increase the problem. One should consult the doctor.

Is driving safe during pregnancy?

One can drive until labour starts. However, during the first month judgement does not remain precise, you should therefore drive cautiously.

Should one continue working in office while pregnant?

Pregnancy is a normal phenomena hence one can continue working till one gets tired or due to distended abdomen it becomes uncomfortable.

What type of footwear should one wear?

Attention to footwear is needed because ligaments of foot becomes lax and tend to stretch. Increasing weight and softening of ligaments easily result in flattening of arches of foot. It may cause permanent injury to the architecture of foot. Hence standing for long periods should be avoided.

Shoes and chappals worn during pregnancy should have flat heel providing satisfactory support.

What type of brassiere will suit a pregnant woman?

A good support is essential. Breasts generally enlarge rapidly in the beginning of pregnancy then again around the 20th week. After the 20th week it remains stable till before delivery. Expecting mothers should buy a new brassiere. It should have strong and fairly wide shoulder straps because if breasts are allowed to sag during pregnancy for lack of adequate support then they may sag permanently.

What are nursing brassiers?

Many types are available to feed the child conviniently. One has detachable flap on each side at the level of the nipple surrounding two inches of breasts. Another style has fastenings on the front where the child can be suckled at the breast without undoing the bra.

Is abdominal support needed during pregnancy?

Abdominal enlargement is not obivious till the 16th week. First the waist line disappears on the sides. Women who have strong abdominal muscles do not need any abdominal support. Their muscles will respond to the need of pregnancy and will return to normal after delivery.

If the muscular discomfort persists, it may be relieved by wearing a light weight elastic abdominal support. Certain women who normally wear some abdominal support will require some support during pregnancy as well. It will not damage the child.

What type of underwear should pregnant woman wear?

Generally Indian women wear petticoats and they can continue wearing these. Girls who wear the type of underwear in the non pregnant state may continue. Tight fitting underwear may be harmful and uncomfortable. Cotton panties in hot weather are comfortable.

Do hair need extra care during pregnancy?

Dry hair tends to become more dry and greasy hair more greasy. So one should use an appropriate shampoo for particular type of hair.

Some ladies loose more hair during pregnancy. Hair becomes thin too. They should not brush too vigorously.

What about nails of pregnant ladies?

In some cases nails become fragile. In some cases nails may

become brittle, crack or break. Brittle nails will break doing household work. Some rub baby oil into base of the nails to check breaking.

What is the effect of smoking in pregnancy?

Heavy smoking is to be discouraged specially during pregnancy. Babies of those who continue heavy smoking after the 16th week may have mental and physical retardation in late childhood. Placenta may reduce oxygen supply depriving nutrition to fetus. Fetus will also be about 250 grams lighter in weight.

What is the effect of alcohol consumption during pregnancy?

Heavy consumption may cause congenital abnormalities. Although there is no evidence that a glass of wine or sherry or beer is harmful but it is advisable to not drink whisky during pregnancy.

What about 'bath' during pregnancy?

One may continue with one's normal bathing habits. But care should be taken to see that the water is not too hot. Also one should not bathe for very long periods. One should take proper care to avoid disbalance due to protruded abdomen while getting in and out of bathroom. Vulva and surrounding area should be washed and dried properly.

Is douching advisable in pregnancy?

Douching is not popular in India. It is not advisable because if more pressure is applied then the water, through the vagina, can enter the uterus and interfere in the continuation of the pregnancy. Antiseptic solutions should never be used.

What type of care do teeth require during pregnancy?

During pregnancy teeth are prone to decay. It is believed that this may be so because some calcium is being utilised by the baby. During pregnancy infection of gums or gingivitis is common because gums become softer and more vascular.

- One should clean the teeth after every meal.
- Use a medium brush. If bleeding occurs, use a soft brush or rinse with mouth wash.

What type of skin care is needed during pregnancy?

There is an increased pigmentation of skin during pregnancy. Specific pigmentation develop on breast and abdomen. Brown unnoticed hair on arms and legs become prominent. Colour of hair may become normal after delivery.

Local areas of irritation may develop. Cleanliness and hygiene has to be maintained.

What type of stretch marks develop during pregnancy?

During pregnancy stretch marks may occur in the abdomen area. These may also appear on breasts. The dark discolouration continues throughout pregnancy but finally fades out leaving silvery thin scars which never fully disappear.

Does skin become dry?

Women who have oily skin find it more oily and women with dry skin have drier skin. Dry skin may cause itching and irritation.

Rubbing a small amount of oil will help.

Is excessive secretion of saliva common in pregnancy?

Excessive salivation of mouth is accompanied with an offensive taste. Women need to spit saliva off and on. Production of saliva is more than 1.5 litres a day. Condition may improve as pregnancy advances but persists till delivery.

Does vaginal irritation take place?

It is always associated with irritation of vulva. Pelvic congestion may further add to the irritation. Infection is caused by bacteria. If discharge has an offensive smell then consult the doctor.

Is monilial infection common?

Pregnant woman is susceptible to the infection of thrush. Soreness and irritation develop . Fungicidal cream helps in treatment.

Why do women develop shortness of breath during pregnancy?

These develop intermittent shortness of breath specially when uterus enlarges and pushes diaphragm upwords in to chest. But it does not incapicitate a woman for day to day work. Shortness of breath becomes marked while lying flat in bed and can be released

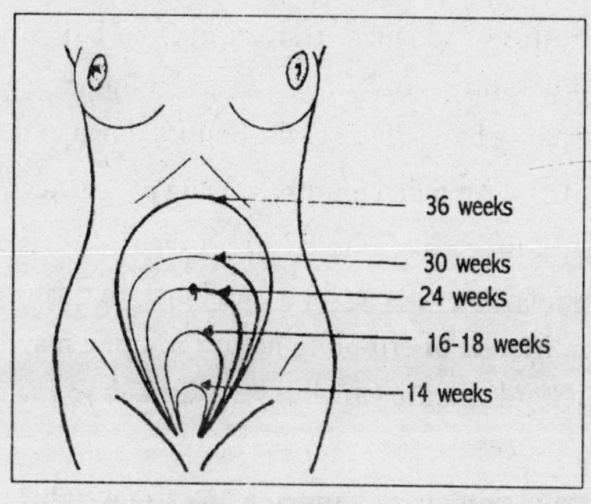

FUNDAL HEIGHT

by raising the head. During the process of delivery when head slides down, pressure on diaphragm is released.

Why do some pregnant women develop a feeling of faintness?

Most pregnant women feel faintness on some occasion during the early days of pregnancy. Fainting develops due to lowering of blood pressure. If blood pressure falls below a certain level the blood supply to the brain is reduced causing faintness. As a woman faints and falls down, the brain comes to a lower ground level and blood supply to brain is automatically restored. It is common during the first 3 months of pregnancy. Actual feeling of faintness is not harmful. Recovery is rapid without harming baby or the mother.

Why some females develop backache during pregnancy?

Backache is a common symptom throughout pregnancy. Progesterone produced by the placenta softens the tendons and ligaments. Characteristic posture of a pregnant woman places a considerable strain on the lower joints of spine. This becomes worst in bad posture. Adequate rest during the last 3 months is of importance. Prolapse of disc involving sciatica nerve results in pain radiating through the centre of the buttock down to the back of leg.

Is sacro-iliac joint pain common during pregnancy?

Sacro iliac joint pain results in low backache. Pain is over the joint and is distinctive. Such pain becomes worse on rotatory movement. This condition is of crippling nature and one may find difficult to walk. Good posture which is very difficult to maintain is to be tried.

Why do some pregnant women gain extra weight?

Excessive weight gain results in backache. So one has to maintain the desired weight throughout the pregnancy. Some develop increased appetite and eat more without doing any physical work and thus gain a lot of excess weight.

Do some pregnant women are prone to developing varicose veins?

Varicose veins may develop in the lower legs in any stage of pregnancy. As pregnancy advances the uterus increases in size pressing on the veins in the pelvis. Obstruction in back flow of blood from legs to heart increases pressure within the veins of the legs. This results in varicosity of veins. Excess weight gain during pregnancy further causes veins to dilate. There is also a hereditory factor in developing varicose vein.

How often does varicosity develops?

It is rare to develop varicosity in the first pregnancy and specially during the first three months. After delivery obstruction due to enlarged uterus is relieved. Varicosity becomes more severe with each pregnancy. Mild varicosity may improve but severe varicosity may regress only partially.

What do varicose veins look like?

Varicose veins first appear as a spiderly network. Affected veins become distended, soft, turgid cords lying beneath the skin. A bluish colouration also develops.

How varicose formation may be prevented?

- Avoid gaining excessive weight.
- Do not stand still for long periods.
- Avoid crossing the legs.
- Do gentle exercise.
- Avoid wearing underwear with any form of elastic band.
- Raise the feet when sitting down .

What are the signs/symptoms of varicosity?

Mild irritation over skin may be the first sign. There may be a disturbing bluish colour. In severe cases skin becomes shiny and thin. In the end it may ulcerate to form varicose ulcer. Dilated veins may cause swelling of ankles and feet. There may develop aching pain specially during night.

Elastic nylon stockings provide support. It assists the venous return. Such elastic support has to be worn throughout the day.

Can vulval varicose veins develop during pregnancy?

Varicosity of veins may develop in the labia majora . These may result in severe aching and irritation. Support for veins is not possible but wearing of sanitary pads may provide relief. During delivery such veins may burst which can be controlled by pressing with finger. Vulval varicose veins usually disappear after delivery.

Can pregnancy lead to piles?

Piles are varicose veins in and around the rectum and anal canal. Piles are caused by

- Progesterone relaxing the smooth muscle of blood vessels.
- Constipation and straining.
- Hereditary predisposition.
- Pressure of baby's head may obstruct the vein.

What are the symptoms of piles?

Presence of hard and bulky faeces passing out with strain result in enlargement of varicose veins. When veins become large these protrude out of the anus. Protrusion occurs momentarily with the passage of motion but later may remain prolapsed. Bleeding occurs separately while passing faecal matter. Local irritation around anus is common. Local soreness and even pain may be present. This painful condition occurs during the 6th to 8th weeks of pregnancy. Local use of proctosedyl ointment will relieve symptoms.

What do you understand by intertrigo during pregnancy?

It is a red irritating skin rash where folds of skin are in close contact. It is mostly seen underneath breasts and also in groin. It is more common in overweight women and is caused by liberal quantity of sweat. One should prevent the skin becoming wet. Putting talcum powder after drying the part will help.

What do you understand by 'linea nigra'?

It is a dark line developing in the centre of abdomen starting around the 14th week of pregnancy. Width of it may be one centimetre. It has no special significance to mother or child. It begins to fade soon after delivery. Pigmentation around umbilicus remains for several years.

What is the butterfly stain on face in pregnancy?

It occurs on face exposed to the sun. It has a butterfly shaped distribution spreading from nose over cheeks like wings of butterfly. It has no special significance. If you bleach, then this will become more obvious. Otherwise this will normally fade a few days after delivery.

Can bleeding from nose take place during pregnancy?

Nose bleeding is transient and small in amount. Mucus membrane of nose has a greatly increased blood supply during pregnancy making it more prone to damage. Nose bleeds should be treated by applying pressure with a handkerchief to the affected nostril or by gently pinching the nose. If nasal passage is dry and cracked a small amount of vaseline can be applied.

Why do pregnant women develop muscle cramps in their legs?

Cramps in calf muscles are more frequent during last three months of pregnancy specially during the night. They can be intensely painful extending from the calf to the foot. Women may suddenly wake up crying out. If she is bent with the toes upwards some relief will be felt. Violent massage will be helpful. Tenderness remains in calf muscles for hours. Cramps are thought to be due to low level of calcium. In some cases it may result due to low sodium content too.

Can costal margin pain develop during pregnancy?

Towards the end of pregnancy the woman may feel pain in her lower chest wall. This is caused by pressure on lower ribs due to the enlarging uterus after 3 weeks of pregnancy. Because the uterus enlarges more on right, pain also develops on that side. Suddenly ribs may become sore and pain may increase. Pain disappears after delivery. Patient is to be reassured.

How do round ligament pain develops?

It is caused by the stretching of the round ligaments of the uterus. It develops between the 16th and the 20th weeks. It is a dragging pain and can be confused with appendicitis. There is no particular treatment except assurance.

Does oedema commonly develop during pregnancy?

It develops due to retention of water in body. Salt is the main source which allows retention of water in the body. Extra amount of water pools down in the foot and ankle due to gravity. Fluid may accumulate due to long periods of standing in hot weather. During the night if the foot is kept raised oedema disappears.

If oedema does not disappear consult your doctor.

A little oedema does not require any treatment but severe oedema in winter can be controlled by a salt free diet and rest during the afternoons. Pickles and papad are to be omitted in the diet.

Why do certain pregnant women develop swelling of face?

Certain amount of swelling of face is common. It is really a fullness of face due to phenomenon. It is also caused by water retention in the body. Diet restriction and giving of diuretics can help.

How do swelling of fingers develop during pregnancy?

Knuckle joints of fingers tend to become much larger. It becomes difficult to take out rings. Otherwise there is no other discomfort. Oedema becomes more pronounced during night. Severe swelling of fingers may occur as a symptom of pre eclampsia. Diet regulation and diuretics can help.

What is the carpal tunnel syndrome?

A pain develops in the wrist and pins and needles can be felt from the wrist down. Carpal tunnel lies in front of the wrist and carries tendons and nerves to the palm. Any swelling results in pressure on tendons and nerves in this tunnel. Pain is more in early hours. There is a stiffness of joints in the hand that's why the patient is not able to hold articles in her hand during the early hours. It always disappears after delivery.

What should a pregnant women do to avoid discomfort in bed?

In the third trimester it becomes very difficult to find a suitable, comfortable position in bed due to protuberant abdomen. Sitting up with 2-3 pillows is the most comfortable position left. Firm bed is required. Heart burn during night hours can also be cured by raising your head.

Why does insomnia develop during the night hours in pregnancy?

Insomnia is the inability to sleep sound specially during the last 3 months. Movements of the baby becomes more vigorous during the night, thus disturbing the sleep pattern. Increased frequency of micturition results in an inability to sleep through the night. The mother has to wake up off and on.

Is cystitis a common problem of pregnancy?

About 25 per cent women develop infection of urinary bladder. They complaint of pain before and after passing the urine. This infection is of a recurrent nature. There will be a rise of temperature with shivering. There will be pain in the kidney area. Suitable antibiotics are available to treat this condition after specific urine culture have been done.

Why do women develop abnormal food desires?

It is known as pica, i.e. a craving for abnormal food, e.g. lemon, tamarind, chalk etc. It used to be an indication of pregnancy in older times.

Pica today is less common. Iron supplements with vitamins may be given.

Pregnancy and Common Diseases

Dr. Mrs. Rati Acharya

What about heart disease in pregnancy?

Commonly output of blood is increased by 30-50% and as a result of this the heart enlarges. Due to enlargement of the abdomen, the heart is pushed up to one side. Mother will note that the heart is beating faster. Palpitation may be unpleasant. Previously termination of pregnancy was advised but these days this condition can be treated and managed.

What if heart disease is diagnosed during antenatal period?

If there are no symptoms other than a slight shortness of breath after exertion, pregnancy will be uncomplicated and there will be no risk to the mother and the child.

If the heart disease is mild, restrictive physical activity is the most effective method to prevent future problems. Anxiety and stress may be avoided.

What about heart diseases and labour?

Generally normal delivery can happen. Even otherwise at the time of delivery an oxygen cylinder may be used to relieve breathlessness or chest pain. Epidural anesthesia can be helpful. Pain and anxiety can be relieved by drugs.

Second stage of labour may be shortened as excessive pushing may cause an added strain on heart. Under such conditions generally forceps are to be applied.

Can heart surgery be done during pregnancy?

In exceptional circumstances heart surgery may be carried out during pregnancy. This is needed when there is a narrowing of valves and the pregnancy may jeopardize the mother's health.

In severe heart disease the pregnancy may have to be terminated at the early stage.

What is the relationship between diabetes and pregnancy?

Diabetes is one of the important causes of infertility. Since the introduction of insulin in 1921 however, the situation has changed. Better investigation and better drugs are available now. Now many women with controlled diabetes are able to become pregnant.

How is diabetes detected in pregnancy?

It may be detected through the presence of excessive sugar in the urine specimen which is tested at the first visit to the antenatal clinic.

Sugar in the urine does not necessarily mean that the woman has diabetes because the pregnancy itself sometimes causes an overload of sugar in the body. Even confirmatory blood tests suggesting diabetes may not mean that the pregnant woman will suffer from diabetes throughout her life. Sometimes stress of pregnancy may produce a diabetic like state which disappears once the baby is born.

What are the chances of the fetus inheriting diabetes?

Educated diabetic mother will always like to know the chances of her son/daughter getting the disease but no definite answer is available.

How to manage diabetes in pregnancy?

Strict control of sugar levels in a pregnant diabetic is important in preventing certain complications in mother and baby. Survival of baby of a diabetic mother wll depend largely on this degree of control. Hence treatment of the mother is to be monitored closely. Previously, in such cases the safe method of delivery used to be a caesarian section. Once born, the child would need extra care.

What can be the effects of diabetes?

- Amniotic fluid may be more. Polyhydramnios (more of amniotic fluid) increases the risk of malpresentation, cord prolapse and inertia.
- Birth asphyxia is more common.
- Shoulder dystocia is a possible hazard. Caesarean section is indicated for diabetes. It is reserved for obstetric indications like large fetus, fetal distress and diabetes which is not under control.

What type of postnatal care is necessary in case of a diabetic?

- Carbohydrate metabolism returns to normal quickly after delivery hence requirement of insulin may fall.
- A diabetic mother who is breast feeding should consume 50 grams of carbohydrates more and adjust the insulin accordingly.
- Small amount of insulin may come in the breast milk but this insulin will be destroyed in the child's stomach.
- A diabetic women is more prone to infections.

What are the clinical features of asymptomatic bacteriuria?

It is a symptom free. There may be a history of frequency and dysuria in recent past. It may persist after delivery. Diabetes predisposes it. It may develop into anaemia, hypertension, preclampsia, preterm labour and low birth baby. Nalidixic acid 400 mg twice a day for 14 days is sufficient. If infection persists Norfloxacin 400 mg for 10 days may be given after consulting the doctor.

Why cystitis is common in pregnancy?

Infection comes from bowel flora, vulval and perianeal region. Catheterization may cause it. Symptoms include frequency, urgency and dysuria. Fever and chills are present. E. Coli is a causative factor. Urine shows turbidity with thick white deposits in bottom with fishy odour. Microscopically centrifused sample shows plenty of pus cells plus a few red cells, bacteria and epithelial cells.

Acute type is associated with higher incidence of abortion, premature labour and intra uterine fetal death. Cepahalosporin 500 mg four times a day for 7 days will help.

What about gonorrhoea in pregnancy?

It is a sexually transmitted disease caused by gonococci. There will be local pain, yellowish pus discharge and frequency of urine. Gonorrhoea must be diagnosed early and treated fully with uroflox 800 mg daily for 3 days.

How to deal with trichomonas vaginalis?

It is caused by a pear shaped protozoan. Infection is caused by sexual intercourse. Symptoms include copious frothy vaginal, greenish yellow discharge with vulval itching. Treatment includes tablet metronidazole 200 mg thrice daily for 7 days at all stages of pregnancy. Vaginal tablet inside vagina may be kept for 6 consecutive nights. Husband has to be simultaneously treated.

Its effect on pregnancy includes premature rupture of membranes, preterm delivery and low birth weight baby.

What do you understand by monilial vaginitis?

It is caused by candida albicans. There will be thick curdy white discharge with intense vulval itching. Vulva will be red and vagina will have curdy flakes on vaginal mucosa. Treatment includes Conestan vaginal tablet 100 mg to be pushed in to the vagina for 6 nights. Course may be repeated if needed. Clotrimazole cream is applied on vulva at bed time.

ANEMIA

When anemia is labelled?

Anemia in pregnancy is decrease of hemoglobin below 10 gram. Vitamin B_{12} and folic acid are essential for synthesis of DNA in haemopoitic cell. Vitamin C helps in absorption of dietary iron and utilization of folic acid. Sufficient amount of protein is required.

What is the lower limit of hemoglobin to be labelled anemia?

Lower limit of physiological anemia is

- RBC upto 3.2 million per cubic millimeter
- Hemoglobin upto 10 gram %
- Hematocrit 32%

There is a need for prophylactic iron therapy to improve physiological anemia.

What are the causes of nutritional anemia?

Inadequate food intake, repeated pregnancies, gastric hyposecretion, low folic acid, infections and haemorrhage results in anemia. Abortions, hookwarm infestations, malaria are more common in India.

How to differentiate between iron deficiency and nutritional macrocytic anemia?

	Iron deficiency anemia	**Nutritional anemia**
Etiology	Deficiency of iron	Deficiency of folic acid or vit. B12
Diarrhoea	+	—
Jaundice	Usually present	Present
Parity	More in high parity	High in low parity
Oedema	+	+
Peripheral neuritis	Absent	Usually not present
Glossitis	In 30%	In 50%
Spleen	Enlarged in 20%	Same size

What are the clinical features of anemia?

Symptoms include asymptomatic fatigue, asthenia, exertional dysponea. There may be swelling of face and feet.

It may result in stillbirth, low birth weight, increased neonatal death and anemia in the baby.

How to treat anemia in pregnancy?

As prophylaxis 200 mg ferrous sulphate a day with meal taken by the pregnant woman after first 3 months of pregnancy and during period of breast feeding is useful.

Addition of 500 mg folic acid a day helps in prevention of folic acid deficiency.

What foods can be helpful in pregnancy?

(i) Food contaning folic acid includes fruits and green vegetables. Milk is poor in folic acid.

(ii) Food containing vitamin B_{12} includes liver and meat. Vegetables don't contain B_{12}. Very little amount is present in egg and milk.

(iii) Food containing iron includes egg, meat, and liver. Vegetable source includes peas, green leaves, lentils, fruits and mollasses.

SYPHILIS

What about syphilis in pregnancy?

Syphilis is caused by treponema palladum. Incubation period is 6 weeks. It is classified into primary, secondary and tertiary.

- In primary lesion papule is followed by ulcer developing on vagina and cervix. It heals in 3 to 6 weeks. In pregnancy it may go unnoticed.
- Secondary lesion appears 6 to 8 weeks after healing of primary lesion as skin rashes on palms and soles.
- Tertiary syphilis may develop at any site.

Treponema palladum spirochete or syphilitic infection affects the placenta and the fetus. In cases of virulent infection abortion occurs. There may be a still birth or macerated fetus may be delivered.

What will be the features of a syphilis infected fetus?

Clinical evidence of syphilis in a baby are snuffling, saddle nose deformity, enlargement of liver, desquamation of skin, flaccid paralysis of leg or arm with a swelling at the end of a long bone.

X-Ray shows osteochondritis or periostitis.

COMMON PROBLEMS OF PREGNANCY

What are fibroids?

These tumors of uterus arise from smooth muscles. These become larger during pregnancy. These are generally multiple and may vary in size from peanuts to a big ball. Atrophy of most fibroid

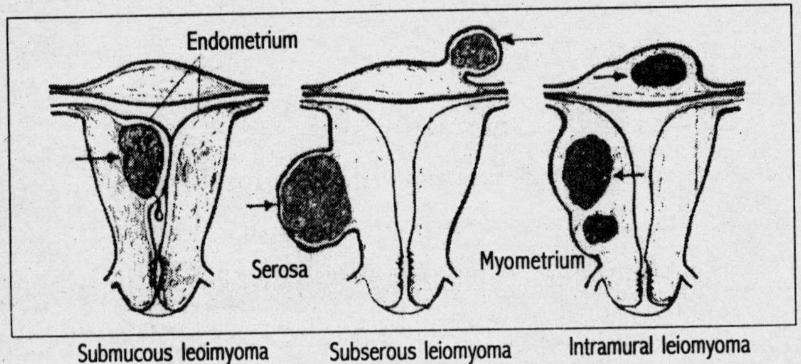

occurs after menopause. Only 0.5% can change into malignancy. Torsion of it may produce pain, shock and vomiting. Bleeding is very common. Abortion may take place with submucus fibroids. Surgical removal is safer.

What do you understand by abortion?

Abortion is the termination of pregnancy before the fetus is capable of surviving outside the uterus.

1. In threatened abortion there is vaginal bleeding before the 20th week of pregnancy. There may be pain in lower abdomen.

2. In inevitable abortion cervix begins to dilate and membranes have already ruptured making it impossible for the pregnancy to continue.
3. In incomplete abortion fetus is expelled but a portion of it is retained in uterus which becomes a source of continuing bleeding.
4. Missed abortion is death of fetus in uterus before the 20th week but products are retained in uterus for a prolonged time. In such cases morning sickness ceases at once and the size of uterus does not grow further.

What are the types of twin pregnancy?

- Non identical twins develop from two separate ova which

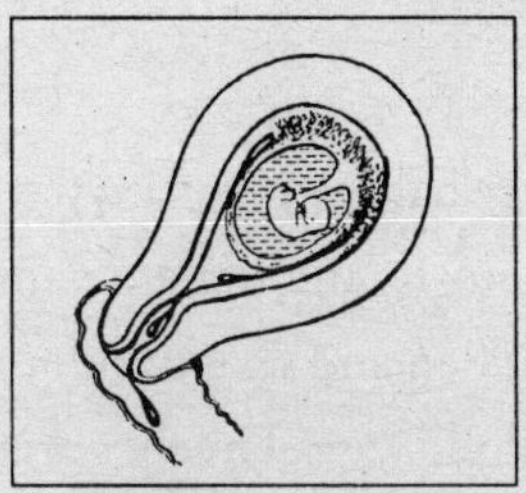

Threatened Abortion

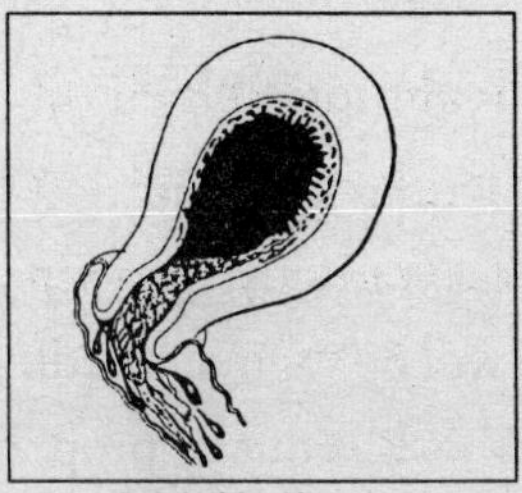

Inevitable Abortion

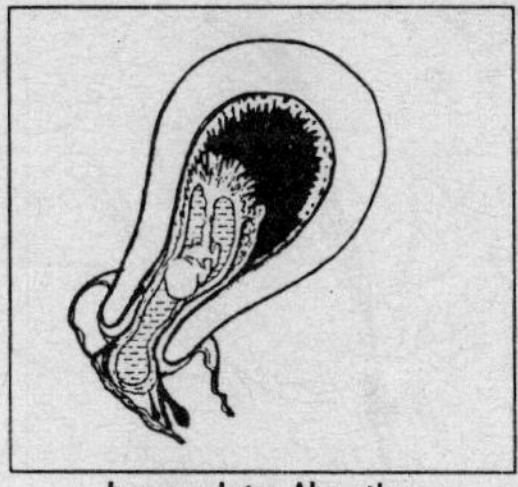

Incomplete Abortion

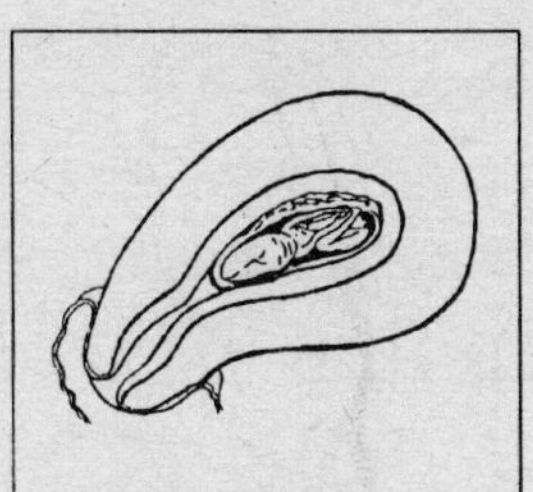

Missed Abortion

may or may not come from the same ovary. There are two separate placentas and their genes differs.

- Identical twins develop from a single ovum which after fertilization undergoes division to form two embroys. These are always of same sex and their genes are identical.

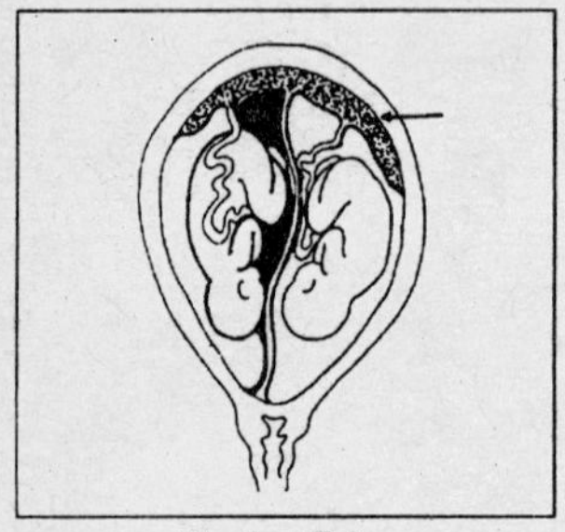

Identical Twins

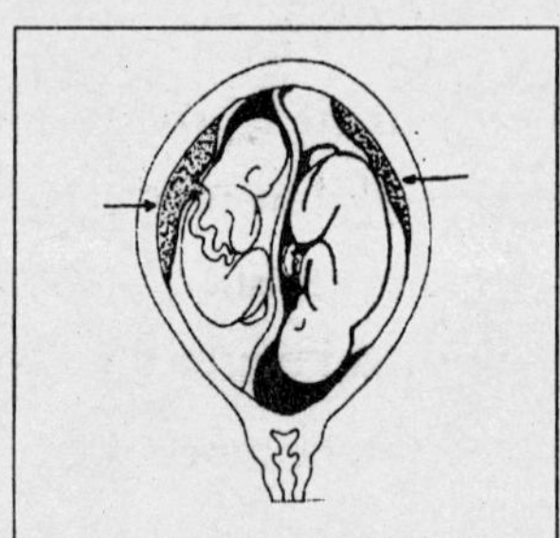

Non Identical Twins

What is abruptio placenta?

It is a serious complication in the later half of pregnancy where the placenta undergoes separation from its uterine attachment. There will be vaginal bleeding with sudden and severe abdominal pain. Shock is out of proportion of blood loss. Timely ceasarian section may help if fetus is alive.

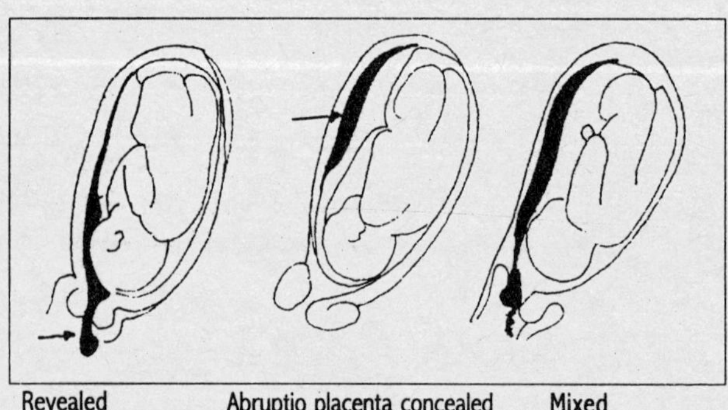

Revealed Abruptio placenta concealed Mixed

What is placenta previa?

It is the development of the placenta in the lower uterine segment so that it partially or totally covers the cervix. It may be complete or incomplete. Painless, bright red bleeding is the feature of it.

How does the prolapse of the cord affect a pregnancy?

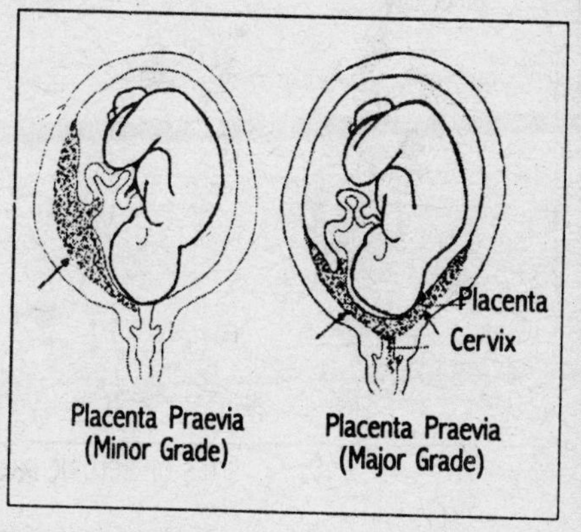

It is a condition in which membranes rupture allowing cord to prolapse through cervix. Cause of it may be (i) Breech presentation (ii) Multiple pregnancy (iii) Polyhydraminos and (iv) Preterm rupture of membrane. This condition has high mortality rate due to cut off of blood supply. Prolapse of cord is of various types.

What is an ectopic pregnancy?

In simple words it is a pregnancy outside the uterus. Bleeding is

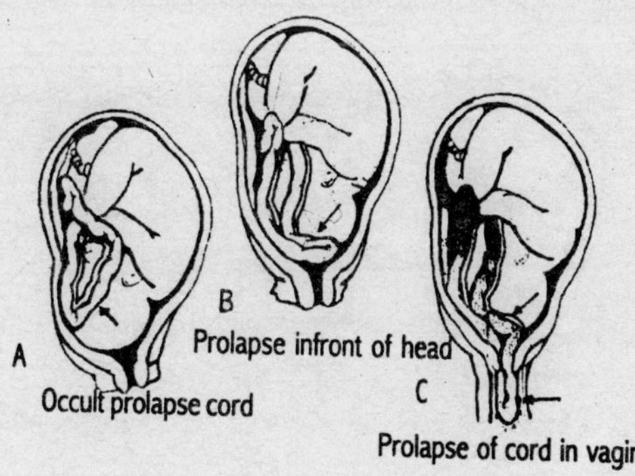

an early symptom. The cause for this is not known. Commonest site involved is fallopian tube. It has a high fetal mortality and requires an early surgery.

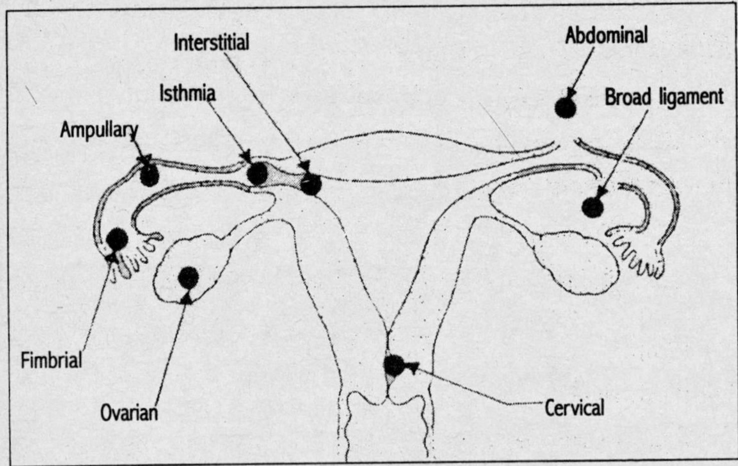

SITES OF ECTOPIC PREGNANCIES

Signs and Stages of Labour

Dr. Sujata

Labour is something special and different for every woman. To pinpoint when it begins and how long it will last is not really possible. For about a month body prepares itself for labour. The cervix dilates and thins out.

What is 'engaging' of the head?

Head of the fetus settles down into the pelvis. At this stage the abdomen will seem lower and will protrude more. One can still breath easily.

Will the pregnant woman pass more of urine at this stage?

Once the head is engaged, she may feel an increase of pressure on her pelvis. It may lead to awkwardness while walking. She will have the urge to pass urine more frequently. In the first pregnancy this is felt more.

What about lower backache?

Lower portion of the body can often cause backache and a crampy pre menstrual feeling. Vaginal secretions may increase in the last week of the pregnancy.

Does the baby move faster in the womb?

As baby grows he runs out of space to move around. He is able to move about eight to twelve times a day and you may feel more frequent bowel movements after 48 hours of labour.

What do you understand by false labour?

For several weeks before the actual delivery you may feel contractions. These contractions soften the cervix and open it up for labour. As a rule it is not genuine labour unless the contractions become regular, last longer and come close together.

What is the difference between true and false labour?

True Labour	False Labour
• Contractions are more felt more in the back	• Felt more in the abdomen
• Contractions become stronger, longer and closer together.	• Contractions don't change in intensity.
• Bloody mucus discharge.	• There is no brown, pink or blood coloured mucus.
• Mucus plug blocks the cervix	• No mucus plug
• Activity affects the intensity of contractions	• Activity does not decrease the contractions

What are the three signs of labour?

Signs of true labour include

- Loss of mucus plug or bloody show.
- Rupture of water bag.
- Regular uterine contractions.

What do you understand by blood show?

It is the passing of small blood stained mucus or brownish blood. It is formed in early pregnancy to close off the cervix to prevent infection. If you discharge any fresh blood like heavy periods, please report immediately to the hospital.

Why does the water bag rupture?

In the womb, the fetus is surrounded by amniotic fluid. Rupture of membranes is most likely to occur during a later stage of labour. It can happen as a sudden gush of liquid flowing down your legs. Longer the period between the rupture of membranes and delivery, more the chances of infection.

What type of uterine contractions take place?

Contractions develop at regular intervals and last from 45 seconds to one minute each. These contractions don't go away on activity. Contractions are like strong menstrual cramps. Contractions are

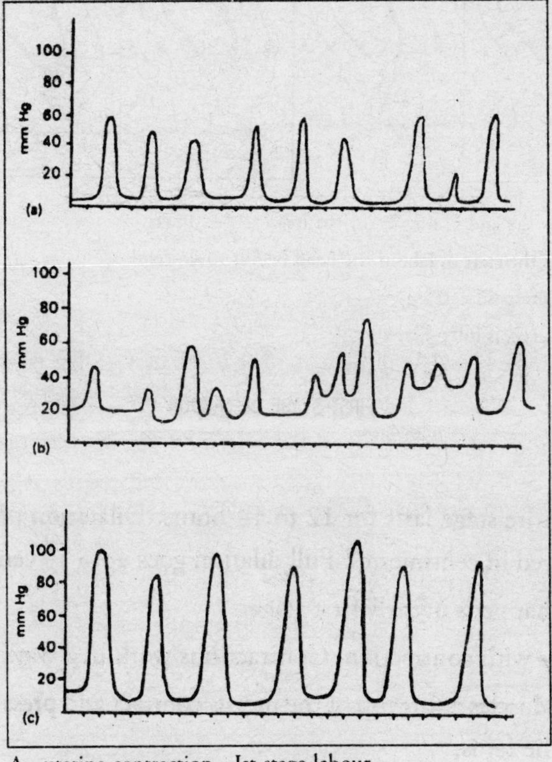

A. uterine contraction - Ist stage labour
C. uterine contraction in primigravida - Ist stage
B. obstructed labour in multigravida

accompanied by hardening of uterus which can be felt by placing the hand over it.

What is the first stage of labour?

First stage of labour is divided into three sections

(i) Early or latent stage

(ii) Active stage

(iii) Transitive stage

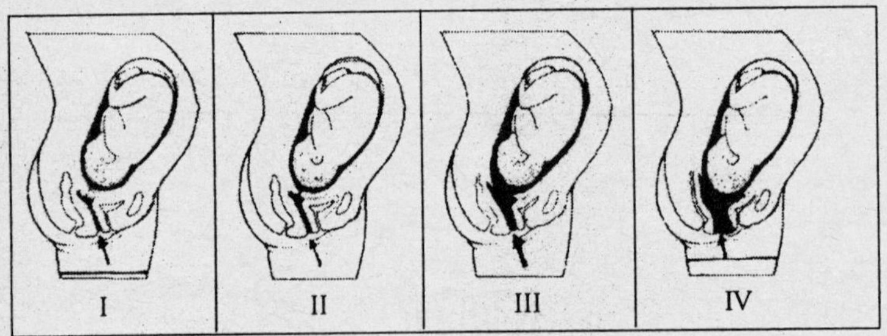

I By the end of pregnancy the head settles down.

II At the start of labour the head begins to descend.

III Cervix dilates.

IV Cervix is fully dilated.

FIRST STAGE OF LABOUR

The entire stage lasts for 12 to 14 hours. Dilatation of cervix is measured in centimetres. Full dilation goes upto 10 centimetres.

What happens in early first stage?

It starts with contraction. Contractions work in 2 ways

(i) Muscles at the top of the uterus contract and press down on the fetus.

(ii) Muscles at the bottom pull upwards making the cervix thin and open.

In this stage cervix opens upto 5 centimetres.

Contractions become more regular and intense.

Some women don't even notice this stage.

What happens in 'active stage'?

In this stage cervix opens from 5 to 8 centimetres. Contractions may develop every 4-5 minutes. This stage lasts from a few minutes to six hours.

What happens in the transition stage?

During this stage woman screams at her husband. She digs her nails hard into her palms. Cervix will dilate from 8 to 10 centimetres. Contractions will come every 60-90 seconds. This stage is the quickest and most intense. It lasts between 15 minutes and 2 hours.

What happens in the second stage?

It begins when the cervix is fully dilated, i.e. 10 centimetres and ends with the birth of the child. The woman may feel like holding her breath. As the head stretches the birth canal and perineum the woman may feel a powerful burning sensation. When the head becomes completely visible at vulva, it is knon as 'crowning'.

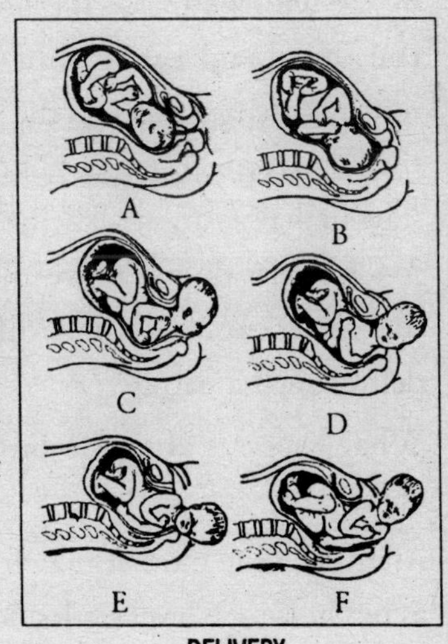

DELIVERY

What is the third stage?

It is the delivery of the placenta. It takes from 15 minutes to half an hour. The woman may be given an injection of hormone. This stimulates the uterus to contract to expel the placenta.

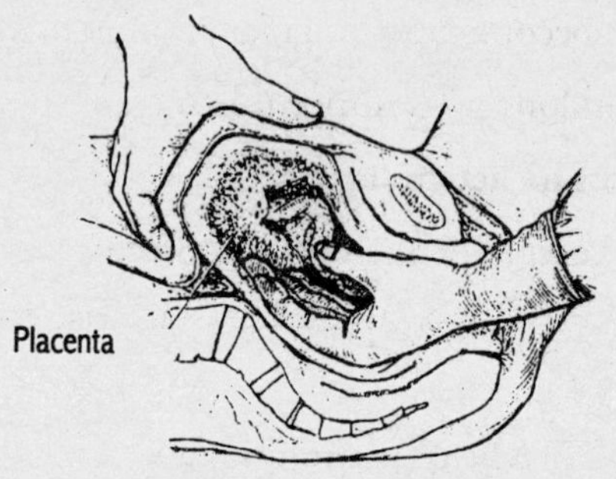

MANUAL REMOVAL OF PLACENTA

What is breech presentation?

During early weeks of pregnancy most of the fetus lie inside the uterus with the head upwards and bottom downwards. But at about the 32nd week the baby turns through half circle and stays in that position till delivery. About 3-4% babies do not move and remain in breech position. It is difficult to deliver such a baby.

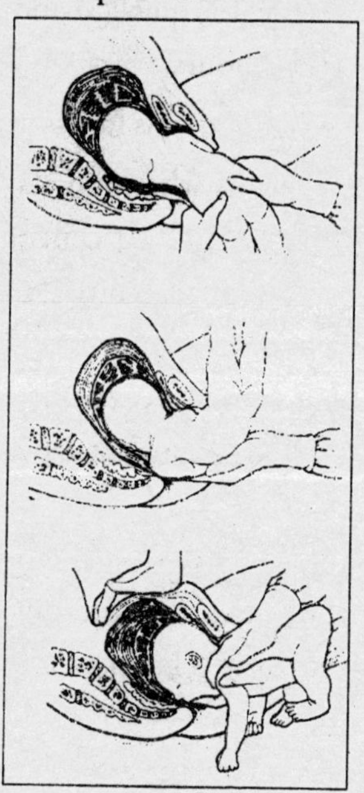

BREECH

What happens after the birth of the child?

After birth the mother may feel weepy as her hormone level settles down. She may feel pain in her abdomen.

When caesarian section needs to be done?

Caesarian operation has to be done when normal delivery is not possible due to the following causes .

- Feto-Pelvic disproportion
- Non progress of labour
- Failed forceps
- Previous caesarian section
- Cancer cervix
- Fetal distress
- Umbilical cord prolapse etc.

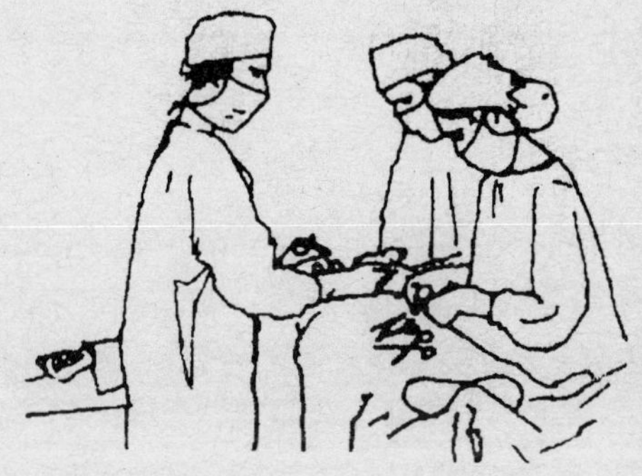

Normal Baby

Dr. Ila Gupta

When the child takes its first breath?

A healthy normal baby starts breathing just after the birth, a pleasurable moment for onlookers. When the baby is inside he relies upon the placenta. He derives oxygen from his mother's blood. The uterus is surrounded by amniotic fluid which he swallows. The baby's lungs remain in collapsed state.

How does respiration starts?

First breath is brought about by response to respiratory centre in the brain. Stimulation to brain comes from the physical contact that the body makes with its surroundings. Other causes include sudden fall in oxygen level after the tying of the umbilical cord, noise, change in temperature etc.

What type of noises does the baby make after birth?

The baby makes strange noises. In response to slightest stimuli he will sneeze quite often. Babies also cough. They develop hicough too.

What is the position of the umbilical cord at birth?

The umbilical cord at birth is pulsating, wet and slippery. Then after the baby starts breathing a clamp is placed on the umbilical cord. Two clamps are put and then the cord is divided between the two clamps. Now the baby becomes a separate entity.

When does the baby cry for the first time?

The baby makes his first cry just after birth. Some cry in full force while others will, cough or splutter. Crying child may become tense and red. Vigorous crying shows that the child is healthy. It completes a full expansion of lungs.

What will be the colour of the new born baby?

When the baby is in the womb his skin is pale yellow. At the time of delivery his colour is pinkish blue. Bluish colour is due to temporary lack of oxygen. As soon as he breaths the colour becomes pink.

On many occasions babies are born in a slightly shocked condition and their colour may be white or pale.

Very frequently new borns will have some fresh blood over their face. An episiotomy or even the slightest laceration may cause it.

What will be the tone of the baby?

The baby is born limp and floppy and has very little or no muscle tone. If child is tense, tone will be of higher degree. Tone of a the baby indicates baby's condition. A limp, flaccid baby will require more of resuscitation.

What is the general appearance of a baby?

The head is big in relation to body. The skull shows gaps where the bones have not fully met, known as fontanelles. There is one in front of the head which generally closes between 12-18 months after birth. Posterior fontanelle is much smaller and can sometimes be felt easily. It closes at 2 months.

What is cephalhematoma?

It occurs due to the stretching of some of veins of the scalp during birth. This collection of blood is harmless and needs no treatment. This disappears between two to three months.

Can forcep delivery also damage skull?

Now a days obstetric forceps are very well designed not to damage skull, still they may leave behind some swelling or slight bruising which fades soon.

What do you understand by lanugo?

Some babies, in addition to scalp black hair, have golden thin hair growing down the back of their necks and across their shoulders. These hair can be rubbed away soon by doing light massage.

What do baby's eyes look like?

Most of the babies are born with bluish eyes but the true colour will appear after sometime only. Generally permanent eye colour is apparent by the time the baby is nine months or so. Hereditary trait plays a great role.

What is vermix?

It is a greasy, yellowish white material seen over the skin of a baby. It is a natural product of his own skin. In the womb it protects the baby.

Can a baby develop jaundice?

Yes, some develop yellowish tinge to the skin and the sclera of eyes just after birth. It is natural and happens due to the natural breakdown of red blood cells. There is no need to worry and it will fade away soon.

What should be the normal length and weight of a baby?

A full term new born baby is 18 to 21 inches long and its weight can vary from 5½ pounds to 10 pounds. Average weight is 7 to 8 pounds. Any baby below 5 pounds is supposed to be a premature child.

What is the position of testicles?

Testicles develop in the abdomen of the baby before birth. Before birth it enters the bag of skin behind the penis called the scrotum. In some cases one or both testicles may stay in the abdomen. Generally in the first month it will come down.

If it does not come down within a year then a doctor should be consulted.

What is a grasp reflex?

If an object is placed across the baby's hand such as pencil or so then baby will immediately grasp it. The baby holds it very tightly. Many muscles work in this process.

What do you understand by 'rooting reflex'?

If anything is put gently on the baby's cheek, he will immediately turn his head to that side. With the help of this reflex the child finds a nipple.

What is 'startle reflex'?

If sharp noise is made the baby will throw out his arms with his hands wide open. Sometimes he will pull his legs up and cry sharply.

Common Birth Defects and Problems

Dr. S. K. Acharya

What is Down's syndrome?

It is also known as Mongolism. The baby's head is smaller than normal and looks flat at the back. Eyes are almond shaped with outer corners facing upwards. Hands are small with square fingers. Little fingers point inwards. Thumb is short. But such a baby is Living and affectionate. Such a child is born to an older primipara. It is not familial.

What is spina bifida?

Literally means split spine. In some cases a swelling is seen. In meningocele swelling may contain of meninges + bag containing fluid.

What is icthiosis?

It is a rare congenital disease. The skin looks like a mosaic design. A baby with this condition may not survive long.

What is hydrocephalus?

In this condition the normal fluid produced in the middle of the brain is in excess. This fluid is known as cerebrospinal fluid. Sometimes surgical interference may be needed.

How does the Apgar score help?

Apgar score takes care of the five physical signs of a baby. Grading is 0, 1, 2 to know how well he is adapting to life outside the womb and whether he has been affected by the process of delivery. The baby is assessed at one minute and five minutes after birth. Score of seven is normal but a baby with low score may be given more care.

Apgar Score

Score	0	1	2
Heart rate	Absent	Less than 100	More than 100
Respiratory effort	Absent	Slow & irregular	Good, regular
Muscle tone	Limp	Flexion of limbs	Active motion
Colour	Blue	Pink body blue extremity	Pink
Reflex response to Catheter	NIL	Grimace	Cough or sneeze

What are the common birth marks?

'Stroke bites' are flat red birth marks. These are found over the bridge of the nose, back of the neck and over the eyelids. Ones which are found over the face generally disappear in one year.

'Mongolian Spots' are irregular areas of deep blue pigmentation. These are found over buttocks.

'Strawberry' marks disappear before the age of five even without treatment.

'Portwine' stains need to be treated with laser therepy.

What are 'Milia spots'?

These are white spots similar to millet seeds. These develop due to distended sweat glands. One finds these over chin, cheeks and nose and are caused by the effect of hormones released from the placenta on the developing sweat glands.

Can infants have enlarged breasts?

Breast enlargement may be seen in many infants but it is of no significance. On occasion even there may be secretion of milk which is due to the effect of hormones from the placenta. There is nothing to worry.

How to test a child's hearing capacity?

It is very difficult to test hearing during first few days because the child is very tolerant of loud noises. Even in the womb he was always hearing noises of bigger artery aorta, gurgling bowel sounds and other things. Still he should respond to a clap or a louder noise.

What about the infant's heart?

Normally an infant's heart beats between 100 to 140 times per minute. Even if some murmurs are heard these may be harmless. If the child becomes blue on playing, he may be examined for 'formen ovale'.

What about first day mucus?

Some children vomit a lot of mucus on the first day and after 24-48 hours. This mucus is produced by the stomach. It is produced in excess quantity for 2-3 days.

Mucus may be very thick thus causing obstruction of respiratory tract resulting in cyanosis. There is no need of special treatment.

Why does babies have sticky eyes?

About 10 to 15% babies develop sticky eyes. One or both eyes start discharging pus or mucus under the lids. At the inner corner of eye there is a tear sac which, in children, gets blocked with a little plug of mucus. Problem will disappear when this plug is cleaned.

One can gently press the fingertips down from the inner corner of the eye to side of the nose, squeezing the fluid from both ends of the tear duct. This has to be done three times a day and ten strokes on each occasion. If eyes become very sticky antibiotic drops may be put. Tear duct massage may be done for few days more even after the problem has been cured.

Why snuffles develop?

It is very common during the first few days. It does not mean that the baby has a cold. If snuffles are interfering with the baby's feeding or sleeping nasal drops can be of help.

Why do babies develop hiccups?

Babies hiccup inside as well as outside the womb. It generally occurs during or after feeds. There is no need to worry and no treatment is required.

What do you understand by pink-stained nappies?

Sometime urine appears to be blood stained. It is not blood but a chemical called urate which babies pass in high quantity for a few days after delivery. It does not require any specific treatment.

Why do babies lose weight during the first few days?

When babies are born their bodies are water logged. They need to get rid of this extra water. Just after delivery for the first 2-3 days no milk or very little amount of milk is produced. This allows him to get rid of some of his water load and moreover he passes urine at normal rate. Child may lose even 10% of his body weight.

Do a few newborns develop fat necrosis?

Yes, a few babies develop rubbery lumps under the skin around the cheek bones. This happens due to rupture of fat cells in skin which sets up an inflammatory reaction. Such lumps will disappear and require no specific treatment.

How is the umbilicus cleaned?

The cord is cleaned regularly at intervals becauses germs grow easily on its surface. One should pull down the gutter and clean with diluted methylated spirit. If the cord gets smelly clean it at regular interval. If the skin around the umbilicus becomes red consult the doctor because it may be due to infection.

Can umbilical hernia take place?

A little swelling may develop under the umbilicus. On increase of abdominal pressure swelling increases and if you squeeze it contents disappear with the sound of gurgling. This hernia does not create any problem. Neither does it burst nor strangulate.

How does nappy rash develop?

The rash occurs in areas of contact with the nappy leaving nappy creases of thigh unaffected. Moisture on the nappy creates irritation of skin. Nappies should be washed in good soap and rinsed carefully. Stop using soap on the skin and instead use a non soap cleanser. Once the rash has improved use a silicone based cream to protect the skin.

What if the child develops rash in a moist area?

This rash tends to be worst in the creases of skin though it may be bad throughout the napkin area.

If rashes are caused by thrush consult the doctor. Some antifungal cream will be helpful.

How to deal with excoriated buttocks?

In some babies rash occurs around the anus and is due to stool. Stool of breast fed babies is very acidic if it is frothy and fluid.

Frequent nappy changing, exposure to air and hydrocortisone creams should improve the condition. A silicon based barrier cream will protect the skin.

Why do some babies develop eczema?

During the first 4 months the skin on the cheeks becomes rough and scaly. In severe form baby can have scaly, cracked, red skin accompanied by weeping. This develops specially over upper body, back of neck and is caused by over activity of sweat glands. It all fades out within the first 6 months.

One should stop using soap for bathing the baby. Avoid using fancy baby lotions.

What do you understand by cradle cap?

Scaliness within hair and eyebrows is known as 'cradle cap'. It responds well to vaseline. Vaseline softens scales and help in those being removed.

What is the rate of bowel action amongst breastfed baby?

There may be 8-10 motions a day or one motion in 3-4 days, all are normal. Breast fed babies have immunity to bacterial gastroenteritis but viral disease can still occur. Stool can be fluidy, seedy or pasty. If he is passing anything other than rabbit pellets, it is normal. Very watery stools like urine is a matter of worry. Loose frequent stools are due to lactose in stool.

What type of stools will be there on bottle feeding?

Bottle fed babies tend to have firmer stools. He may pass stool 4 times a day or once in two days. Colour of stools may be green. If the stool is very firm and hard then well diluted orange juice will be helpful. Loose watery stools in bottle fed babies are risky and doctor may be consulted.

Can a newborn child be taken in air plane?

There is no harm in travelling by flight if the child does not have any lung deformity and has not been born premature. Actually

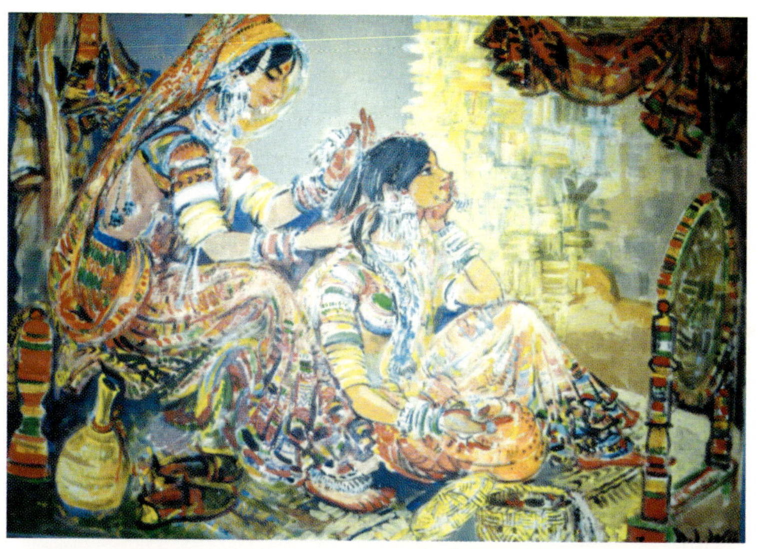

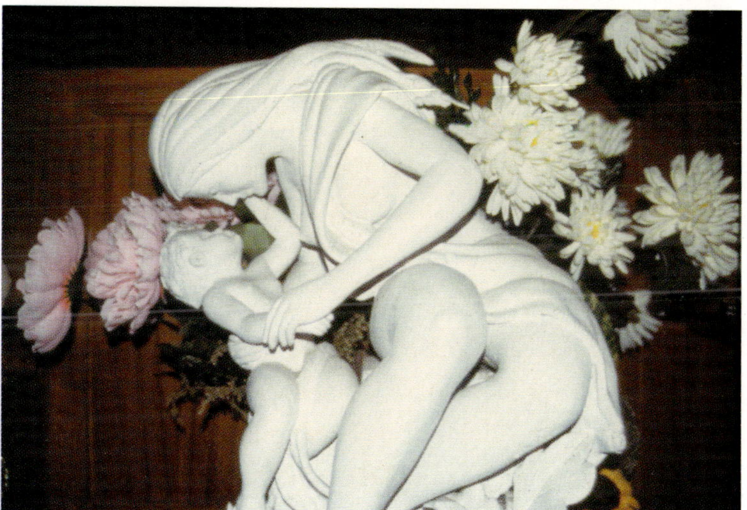

'Mother & child' has been a popular theme for worldclass artists, sculpturists and poets through out the world.

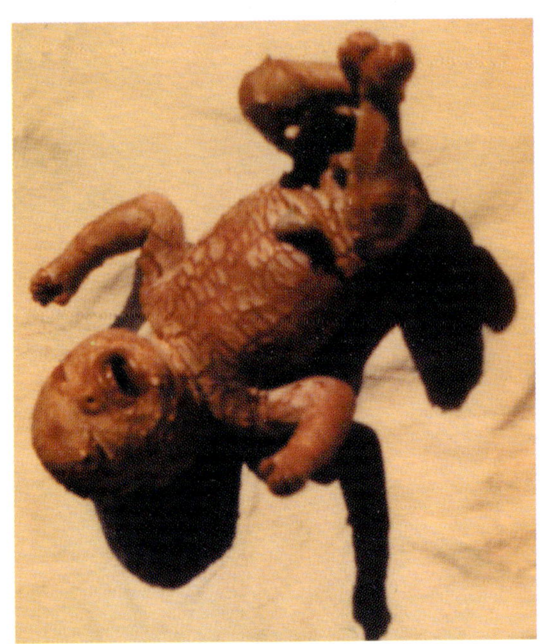

Icthiosis

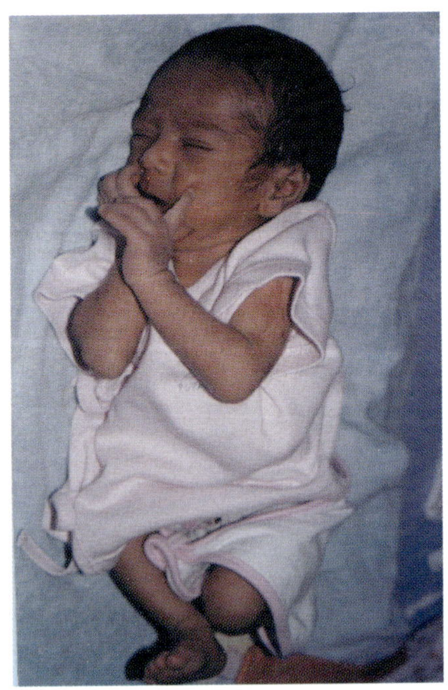

Premature Child

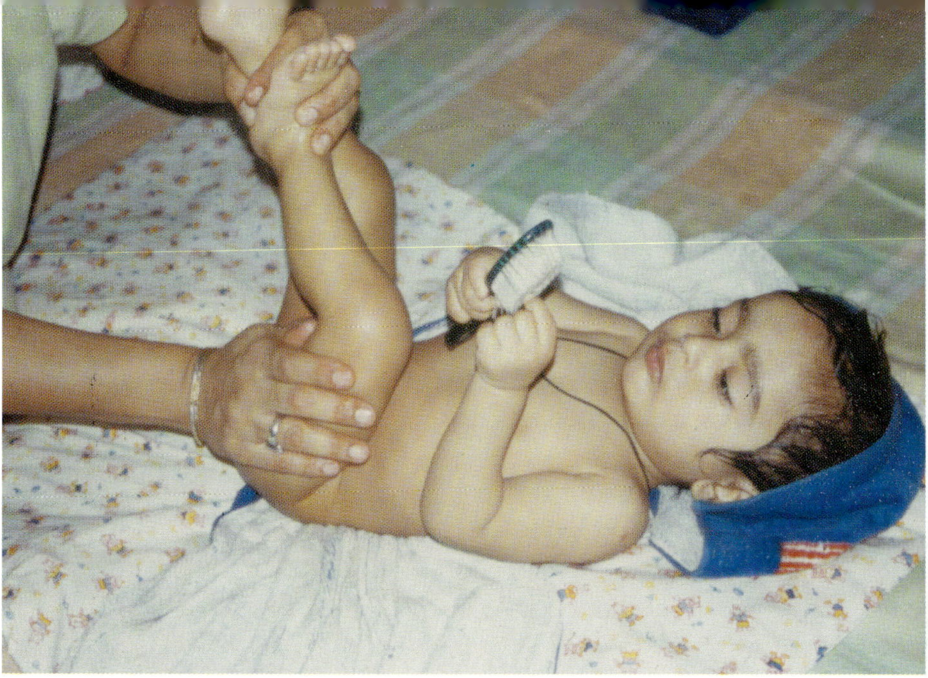

Massage improves blood circulation of body.

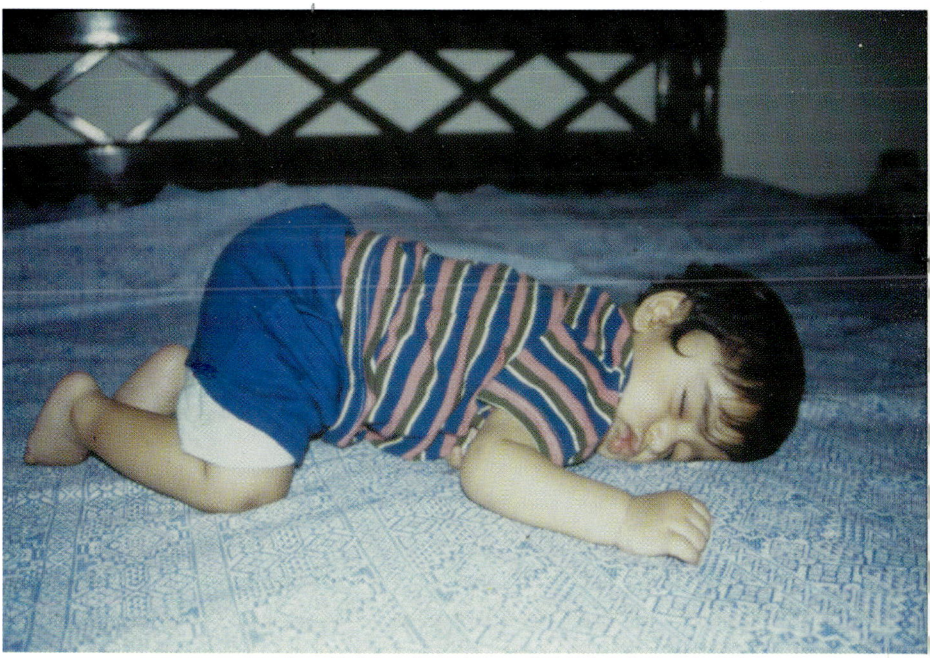

Sound sleep brings freshness.

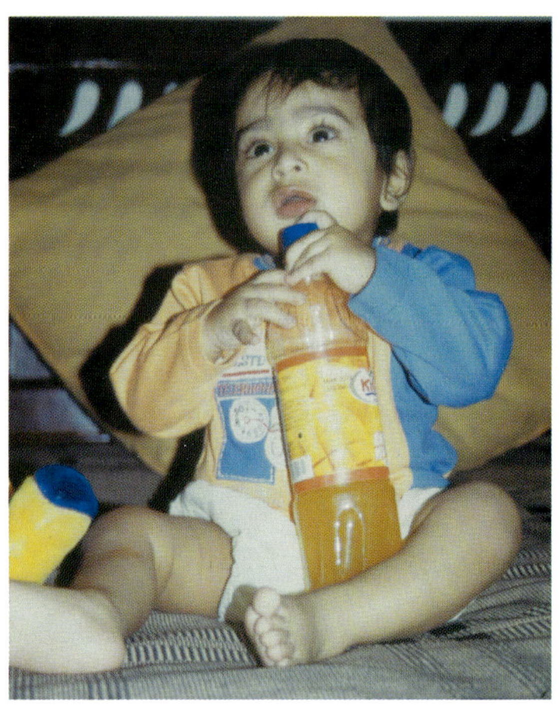

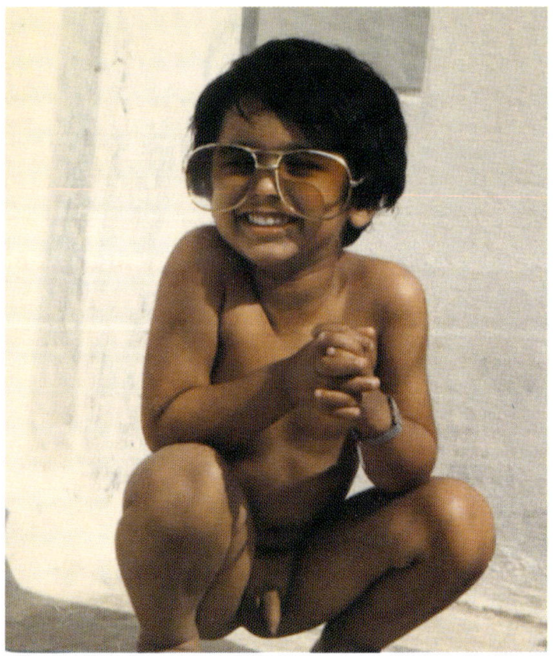

Children are fond of soft drinks and spects.

speaking it is easier to travel with a newborn than a toddler. A toddler will kick left and right and will spill every drink handed over to him.

Pressure problem in middle ear during descending is less common in babies than in adults. It is a good idea to let the baby suck on something when the plane descends as this will equalize the pressure around the ear drum.

How to clean the foreskin?

Foreskin is the skin covering the penis. Foreskin is large enough to let baby's urine out and is not enough to protect the opening of the penis. This skin separates out as the baby grows. For full separation it takes about 3 years. Routine washing even without pulling out the skin will keep the skin neat and clean. At the end of the skin lies a waxy material known as smegma.

Is circumcision advisable of an infant?

Yes, circumscision is the process of cutting off the foreskin. It leaves the head of the penis exposed. In Muslims and Jews circumcision has a religious importance. Previously it was thought that smegma may lead to cancer.

To avoid pain to the baby local anaesthesia may be used. Babies recover within 28 hours of such an operation.

What about the bathing of a newborn?

Bathing newborn just after birth is not a must. Bathing, if not done properly, may cause more harm as it may result in hypothermia. Child may cry vigorously increasing his oxygen consumption.

Following precautions may be taken –

- Excessive vermix may be removed.

- Mother and child care workers should have clean hands.
- First bath should be delayed until vital signs become stable for several hours.
- Preterm baby should be bathed in luke warm water.
- Rubbing and scrubbing may be avoided so that the skin is not injured.

What about taking the baby for a journey?

All children are to be mentally prepared to remain strapped into their seats all the time. Back doors should have a child proof locks.

Always keep one window partly open to ensure fresh air. If you are going on long journey a couple should stop for leg stretching and feed the baby.

Never leave a child alone in a car with its automatic keys. He may press the keys by mistake and car may be closed leaving a child in a miserable condition.

> Being a mother is not just giving a birth to a child but to rear a good human being, a responsible citizen and a good social being.

Breast Feeding

Dr. Ila Gupta

On what factors do the shape and size of breasts depend?

The shape and size depends upon the amount of fat deposited around lobes and lobules and the quality of cooper's ligament. At adolescent woman's breasts are firm and conical. As she grows older breasts become soft and flabby and may sag.

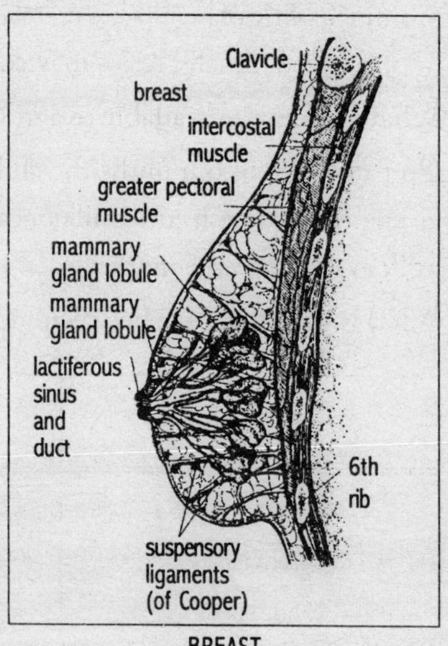

BREAST

Describe the anatomy of breasts?

A girl's breasts develop due to sex hormones secreted by ovaries. Each lactiferous duct system forms a lobe of breast. Lobes are separated by ligaments. Ligaments reach from fibrous tissue which underlies the breasts covering chest muscles, to the layer of fibrous tissue attached to the skin.

Lobes divide into lobules. Then lobules divide further and each lobule is made up of 30 to 100 milk producing alveoli.

What changes takes place during menstruation?

In the first half of the cycle estrogen leads to a growth of ductules and alveoli. During mid period progesterone further increases its growth. Some woman's breast may enlarge from 8 to 20% a week before menstruation. Breasts become tender and heavier. Breasts may be felt nodular.

What changes in breasts take place in pregnancy?

Enlargement takes place due to oestrogen and progesterone increasing throughout pregnancy. Oestrogen makes milk ducts grow and branch while progesterone induces growth of milk producing cells in the alveoli. Hormones increase the size of blood vessels supplying the breasts. Dilated veins beneath the skin becomes prominent. Size of breasts has no relationship with a woman's ability to breast feed. Small breasts may contain more milk.

What options are available to a mother?

Up to the age of 6 months the child can be breast fed or can be given modified fresh cow's milk or can be fed artificially on formula milk available in the market.

What is the difference between mother's and cow's milk?

	Human Milk	Cow's Milk
Protein gm/100 ml	0.9	3.3
Casein %	20	82
Whey %	80	18
Fat gm/100 ml	4.5	3.7
Milk sugar – lactose	6.8	4.8
Calcium mg/100 ml	34	124
Phosphorus mg/100 ml	14	96
Sodium mmol/litre	7	25
Vitamin A I.U./100 ml	190	100
Vitamin B1 I.U./100 ml	16	44
Vitamin C mg/100 ml	43	11
Calories/100 ml	75	69

What should be the interval between two feeds?

Breast fed babies whose stomach empty more quickly are to be fed every 2-3 hours while bottle fed babies are to be fed at the interval of 3-4 hours.

In what way human milk is better?

(i) Human milk curd is soft and floculent containing a high proportion of whey which helps child absorb milk protein easily.

(ii) Human milk contains more of milk lactose than cow's milk.

(iii) Lactose of human milk is a ready source of energy and helps in calcium absorption by baby.

(iv) Proteins of whey contains anti infective substances.

(v) Lactose promotes multiplication of bacteria in the gut of the baby.

(vi) Bacteria produces a weak acid which discourages the bacteria causing gastroenteritis.

(vii) Human and cow's milk contain near about the same quantity of iron but babies absorb more iron from breast milk. About 50% iron is absorbed from a mother's milk and 10% from cow's milk.

(viii) Cow's milk contains more fat. But as fat is less easily absorbed by the body this milk provides less energy.

(ix) Human milk contains lipase which helps in absorption of fat. Lipase breaks down fats releasing fatty acids in the baby's intestine so that fats are partially digested before being absorbed.

(x) Cow's milk contains a higher level of phosphorus than human milk. Phosphorus competes with calcium to be absorbed.

What can be the benefits of breast feeding to the mother?

Breast feeding increases the interaction between mother and her baby. It helps in the development of the child's behaviour.

(ii) Breast feeding improves the skill of mothering.

(iii) Breast feeding mother regains the figure soon.

(iv) Breast feeding is more convinient.

What about mother-baby interaction?

Just after birth when the baby is given to a mother, he learns to recognise her touch, her smell and most probably her face. Such baby cries less and develop night sleep pattern soon.

Is there any relationship between breast feeding and erotic experience?

Yes, erotic experience is increased by skin to skin contact as baby fiddles the breast. Nipple engorges to make it erect similar to when genitals are stimulated directly or in fantasy. There is hardly any difference between child's suckling and lover's sucking.

Mothers who breast feed have an earlier and stronger return of sexual desire. During breast feeding mother touches child, kisses him and adjust her body to provide comfort to the child. This process increases emotional contact.

How does restoration of body figure takes place?

During pregnancy most of women gain at least 3-4 kilograms of body weight. And every woman wants to regain her original figure. Breast feeding women will use up the stored energy sooner than non-breast feeding women.

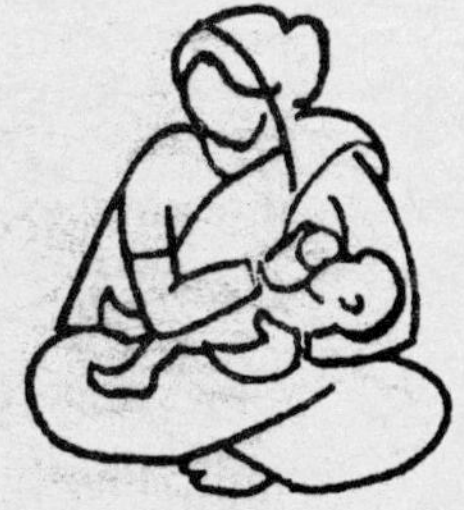

Is breast feeding more convinient?

It is obivious. The mother does not need to clean, sterilize and store feeding bottles.

There is no need to prepare formula milk and to heat it to a suitable temperature.

Human milk is a ready to serve convinient food.

When and how does initiation of lactation starts?

Gland tissue of breasts reaches its maximum by the middle of pregnancy. But milk is not produced until after the delivery of baby when prolactin starts acting on milk producing alveolar cells. Within 2 days of birth of baby blood levels of estrogen and progesteron falls sufficiently to enable prolactin to secrete milk. Breasts become heavier and fuller.

As a baby suckles more, more prolactin is secreted and more milk is produced. Suckling/stimulation of nipple provokes messages along the nerves to the brain where they result in release of prolactin.

What factors influence prolactin reflex?

The mother may be anxious about her ability to feed or may become embarrassed about exposing her breasts. She may find this process a little painful to start. Once lactation has started the alveolar cells secrete milk continuously. Mother may give 200 ml at each feed.

What do you understand by 'let down reflex'?

Milk is of no value unless it is ejected out from alveoli. Milk ejection or let down reflex works in this way. Milk producing alveoli are surrounded by muscle fibres which when contracted squeeze the milk out of sac and propel it along the branching ducts passing to the nipple.

How is the let down reflex initiated?

It is initiated by nerve impulses going to the brain from the nipple due to suckling. It reaches pituitary gland secreting a hormone oxytocin. Oxytocin is released in the blood stream which contracts the tiny muscles network squeezing the milk out. Let down reflex is hindered or helped out by psychological state of mind.

Does poor suckling have any effects?

(i) Poor suckling reduces the poor prolactin reflex and distension of nuclei reduces secretion of milk. (ii) Poor suckling also reduces the release of oxytocin to start 'let down reflex'.

As a result the child cries and the mother looses confidence. She may start thinking that she has insufficient milk.

How to take care of nipple during pregnancy?

Generally during pregnancy nipples become protractile and areola develops. When the woman bathes she should start washing her nipples but not with soaps. Some oil may be rubbed after drying the nipples.

What are inverted nipples?

Generally nipples fit into the mouth of the baby. But sometimes nipples are not fully protractile and are more adherent to the underlying structure. Baby while suckling breaks the adhesions which is painful.

What is pseudo inversion?

A woman can tell if she is has pseudo inversion of nipples. 'Thumb test' can diagnose pseudo inverted nipples. Nipple looks normal but when she presses the edge of areola between her fingers and thumb, instead of nipple remaining protractile it retracts into breast tissue.

Can any exercise help in pseudo inversion of nipple?

She can do specific exercises in the second half of pregnancy to break the adhesions. She should place her opposing thumbs, one on each side of her nipples and draw an areola by moving her thumbs outward. She may do so several times a day. Gentle sucking by the husband during foreplay can also help.

How to learn to breast feed successfully?

Successful breast feeding is learned by watching someone else feeding the child and then by practice. One may follow the procedure of

- Be relaxed and happy. Look and touch your baby.
- Make sure that you are comfortable whether in bed with pillow behind you and one under your knees or lying on side in bed. One may sit on chair putting one's feet up.
- Keep child's arms and hands free to explore, to touch breast.
- Cuddle him so that the child may recognise your smell and touch and start suckling.
- Baby's mouth must be right over the nipple and on areola. Child must be able to breath while sucking.
- Don't force him if he is not hungry.
- Both breasts should be offered to your baby at each feed.

What is 'demand feeding'?

Feeding the baby at request is known as demand feeding. The baby knows well when he is hungry. Some babies need to be fed every 3-4 hours including during night hours while many want to be fed more frequently. But babies who want to be fed more frequently are not sick or under fed. To begin with, the mother should adjust to his need and slowly the baby will learn to adjust to the mother's convinience.

What should be the feeding schedule?

Feeding should not be too rigid. During first few days after birth small amounts of milk is sufficient for the baby. There should be feeding on demand but if child does not ask for more than 3 hours, he may be fed. There should be atleast two night feeds. Child can digest breast milk within 1½ to 2 hours.

What about mid night feeds?

Many babies demand a mid night feed during early life. How so ever it may be inconvinient the mother should meet the demand. If the mother delays the last feed of the day by one hour child may sleep for a longer time.

Can breast milk be stored?

Yes, specially when the mother is a working woman. Breast milk can be kept in refrigerator up to 24 hours and at temperature -20^{0}C can be frozen for 6 months. Milk may not be kept at room temperature for long.

Can breast milk production be increased?

Yes, the mother should consume a nutritious diet

- She should consume a lot of water and milk.
- Massage the breasts slightly.
- Be confident and optimistic and let child play with your breasts.

How long should breast feeding be continued?

It should be continued for 6 to 8 months. Breast milk provides all the nutrients needed by a child. There is no need to add any solids before 4 months of age.

After that the child may be given mashed banana or mashed

portions of food eaten by the family. Of course, the food should be without chillies.

At the age of 6 months the baby's chewing mechanism and digestestive system matures and he starts liking semisolids, which can begin to replace exclusive breast feeding.

Are breast milk banks possible?

Human-milk banks have been set up in some bigger hospitals of the world. This milk is donated by other breast feeding mothers. This milk is meant for preterm babies.

How breast milk can be collected?

Donated milk is hand expressed. Milk is collected, pooled, pasteurized and frozen. But pasteurization eliminates the anti-infective agent in human milk.

What is colostrum?

It is a thick lemon yellow liquid which begins to be secreted in the breasts and may leak from nipples. Colostrum contains less fat, less milk sugar, more protein and a high level of anti-infective substances. It may also be a laxative.

Will smaller breasts produce less milk?

Most pregnant women's breasts reach their maximum size at 20 weeks although there is no relationship between the size of breasts before pregnancy and amount of enlargement during pregnancy. Size of woman's breasts before pregnancy or at childbirth bears no relationship to the amount of milk produced.

Is complete emptying of breasts during feeding necessary?

It is better if breasts empty after feeding. Breasts may be expressed after each feed stimulating lactation and engorgement.

Will breast feeding affect your body figure?

Most women tend to think so. Breasts sag after second or third delivery or if breasts are allowed to become engorged. Once the breasts have sagged nothing much can be done. Creams are of no value although every woman gets some fat deposits during pregnancy. Breast feeding uses some of the deposited fat thus helping a woman to come to her original shape.

How can cracked nipples affect breast feeding?

Baby may be taken off the breasts for 24 hours if nipple is tender and for 2-3 days if cracked. The milk may be expressed from the breasts manually or by breast pump. Lanolin cream may be used.

What can be the difficulties in breast feeding due to the baby?

- If baby is having a cleft palate.
- Premature babies may be too weak to suckle at breasts.
- Thrush infection of mouth may make suckling difficult.
- Nasal congestion.
- Mental abnormality.
- Jaundice causes lethargy and disinclination to feed.

What are the contraindications of breasts feeding?

- Though HIV transmission occurs through breast milk still WHO recommends breast-feeding.
- Maternal psychosis.
- Mothers addicted to drugs or alcohol.
- Certain inborn errors of metabolism e.g. phenylketonuria, glactosemia and alactasia.

How to decide that the child is getting enough feed?

- Child gains 500 grams per month, i.e. about 20 grams daily.

Although during the first few weeks the child will loose weight. Child may be weighed after 2-3 weeks.

- Baby appears healthy.
- Baby passed light coloured urine 6-8 times.

Can some drugs increase breast milk?

Yes, certain drugs have been reported to increase breast milk but frequent suckling is the best. Metachlorpromide is believed to enhance the milk secretion.

What do you understand by 'three month colic'?

Most of the babies during the first three months scream drawing their legs up. The child's face becomes red and he passes wind out of his bottom. Crying is due to colic which generally takes place during evening hours.

Do babies suffer from anxiety?

Anxiety is perceived by baby who becomes more conscious. Although such anxiety can be reduced if the mother picks up her baby, cuddles him, kisses him and reassures that he is being loved.

How does a baby express his hunger?

The baby cries and continues to scream. Even cuddling does not silent him. He stops crying if he can suck at a breast.

What do you understand by 'reflux'?

When some of milk along with acid leaks upwards into the lowest park of esophagus, the child cries. It causes him irritation.

Why do babies pass a lot of wind?

Screaming babies often pass wind from their gut. Screaming builds up the abdominal pressure and air is forced out of the anus. Not passing wind causes colic.

Does breast feeding protect a child from dental carries?

Yes, but how it protects is not clear. It may be that the fluoride content of breast milk is greater. Formula milk has more sugar and may cause dental caries. Another suggestion is that higher selenium content of breast milk is a protective factor.

Can bottle feeding result in dental malocclusion?

Bottle fed babies push their tongues to control the amount of milk and may result in malocclusion. During breast feeding the baby receives more stimulation and uses more muscles than a bottle fed baby. This may be a factor in dental malocclusion.

Will dieting reduce the breast milk?

Crash on quick weight loss diets should be avoided. But if diet is of more than 1500 kcal and the carbohydrate content is more than 100 gm there should not be reduction in breast milk.

Can a woman take every type of drugs during breast feeding?

When a woman is breast feeding she should avoid unnecessary drugs, because certain drugs are excreted in breast milk.

Can the mother take addictive narcotics or alcohol?

Addictive narcotics may cause addiction and severe withdrawls in the baby.

While alcohol in small amounts may be safe, higher amount of alcohol may affect the development of the baby by damaging the nerve connections which are still forming in his brain.

What type of antibiotics should not be taken by the mother?

- Chloromycetin may destroy the baby's white cells.
- Furadantin used to treat urinary tract infection may result in some enzyme deficiency resulting in anemia and jaundice.

- Streptomycin – It may reach in high concentration while treating T.B. This may damage baby's hearing.
- Tetracyclines – It may become incorporated into baby's teeth causing damage to the dentine.

Can the mother use barbiturates?

It is best to be avoided. Large dose may cause drowsiness in baby.

Can the mother take laxatives?

These should be avoided as they are secreted into breast milk and may cause colic and diarrhoea to the child. Senna is safe if taken.

What may be the cause of child's episodic crying?

- Check if child is hungry.
- Check if he is wet, if so then change him.
- Check if he is bored, then cuddle him.
- If he has got wind, help him to pass it.

What is the difference between a complementary and a supplementary feed?

Complementary feed is one in which the formula milk is given to complement the insufficient amount of breast feed. While supplementary feed is a formula feed given in place of a breast feed.

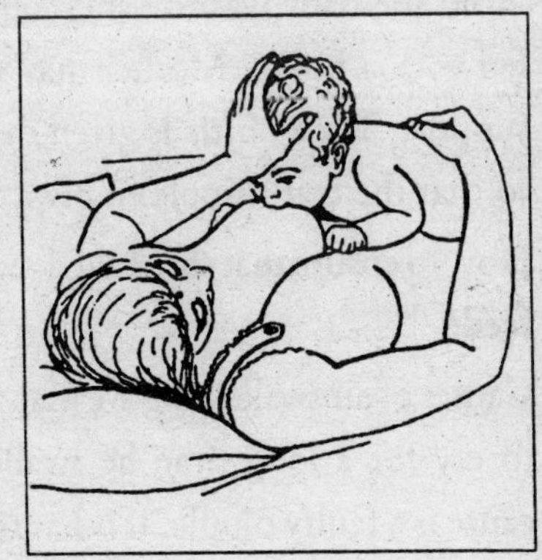

Why do some babies fight with the breasts?

It may be due to frustration when breasts are full and child is not able to get the nipples. Under such circumstances mother may express a little milk manually and then start feeding.

If mother does not support her breast and the breast falls over the baby's nose it may suffocate and he may start fighting with the breast.

Some babies play with the breasts instead of fighting while feeding.

What is formula feeding?

Bottle feeding uses formula milk. Formula milk is based on cow's milk in a modified way. It could be condensed milk, evaporated milk or dry powdered milk. Cheapest formula milk may be lacking essential fatty acids which is disadvantageous to the mental development of the child.

Sweetened condensed milk is lacking in vitamin A.

How to prepare formula milk?

Cleanliness of the highest order has to be maintained. One should ensure that no contamination occurs. Spoon and measuring bottle should be properly boiled before use. Again after feeding, bottle and teats should be boiled for 10 minutes at least. Then prepare milk as per instructions.

What is the technique of bottle feeding?

Hold the baby warmly and comfortably in the arm while being fed with a bottle. Mother may sit comfortably with a firm back support. Then bottle is given to child with a marked upward tilt so that the teat (nipple) is always full of milk at all the time.

How to ensure that the child does not swallow too much air during feed?

Causes of air swallowing are many. When hungry if baby is allowed to cry for a long time he swallows air during crying. Another cause is a faulty nipple. If it has too small a hole the milk passes so slowly that the baby swallows air with it. If the hole is too big then he gulps the milk and along with it.

Best teat is the one made of firm rubber with three small holes. Teats are to be replaced frequently. If teat has become too soft it flattens in baby's mouth creating a vacuum so that child sucks more of air.

How to check that teat is not blocked?

When feed is given with bottle you should not rinse when he is sucking. If bubbles don't subside then take out the bottle from his mouth and make sure it is not blocked by shaking. If it is blocked then change it.

How does one do hand expression?

- Cup breasts in your hand, use right hand for your left breasts.
- Put your thumb above the nipple at the areola and your finger under the nipple at the edge of areola.
- One can feel little bumpy areas where milk has collected in milk duct reservoirs.
- Press your fingers inwards and outwords towards your chest with finger and thumb and rotate your hand so that reservoirs are squeezed.
- The intermittent squeezing leads to milk squirting from nipples which can be collected in a clean container.
- When engorgement becomes less then it can be offered to baby.

When to feed a child?

There are two possibilities

(i) To train the child to accept feed when it suits to mother.

(ii) To allow the child to choose for himself when he wants to be fed.

Demand feeding is when the baby cries and is hungry, then he is put to breast irrespective of time elapsed between two feeds.

What points are to be noted down while preparing baby feeds?

- Don't microwave the feeds.
- Discard the left over feed.
- Use the dried feed within a month once you open the tin.
- Don't add cereals, salt or sugar to feed.
- Use refrigerated feeds within 24 hours.
- Feed the milk warmed either by room temperature or by putting bottle in warm water for a while.
- Don't use tap water to prepare feed.

Can cow's milk be given to a child?

Till 6 months either breast milk or baby milk is suitable. Cow's milk is better after one year of age being low in some essential vitamins such as vitamin A, D and iron. Semi skimmed milk may be used once baby is 2 years of age.

Can several feeds be prepared at a time?

It will be better if feed is prepared fresh on each occasion. Otherwise one can prepare the feed for the whole day and keep it in the refrigerator. But it should be used within 24 hours.

Do breast fed children need iron supplements?

Mother's milk is poor in iron. Baby needs iron to increase hemoglobin in its increasing blood volume and for increasing muscle mass. Amount required may be 0.5-1 mg of iron per litre. Only 40 to 50% of this iron is absorbed into the baby's blood. After 4 months some iron drops may be given intermittently.

What is a physiological jaundice?

In the body there is a constant breakdown and renewal of RBCS. This breakdown accumulates bilirubin in blood. Bilirubin is acted on by an enzyme glucuronyl transpranse and excreted in urine. If too much bilirubin is formed jaundice may result.

Can breast milk cause jaundice in the early stage?

In a few cases a substance known as pregnanediol is excreted in the mother's milk. Pregnanediol does not permit enzyme to act on bilirubin. Hence the baby may become jaundiced when he is of seven days. This may persist for a few weeks. But breast feeding may be continued.

What is the difference between lactation and breast feeding?

While breast feeding includes lactation and interaction between mother and baby and other related problems.

Lactation is the physiological process of secretion of milk.

What are the common causes of jaundice in a new born?

Common causes include –

- Physiological jaundice.
- Blood incompatibility.
- Septicemia.
- Intrauterine infections.
- Breast milk jaundice.

What is a pathological jaundice?

Pathological jaundice refers to jaundice in newborn appearing within 24 hours of delivery and may persist for 14 days. Under such circumstances it is better to consult the doctor.

Can lactation be suppressed?

Many women choose not to breast feed or having started stop it suddenly. There are two available methods.

(1) Just to stop breast feeding. As a result of it breasts become engorged with milk. Pressure of the secreted milk prevents more milk. Also, without sucking the prolactin reflex either ceases or decreases milk production.

(2) Continued milk secretion depends on prolactin reflex. Drugs preventing secretion will reduce production of milk. Until bromocriptine became available estrogen was used for this purpose.

Can breast feeding be continued during menstruation?

Menstruation is not a reason for stopping breast feeding. It has no effect on quality or quantity of breast milk.

Can a woman continue breast feeding if she becomes pregnant again?

Yes she can continue to breast feed. It will not damage her fetus or deprive it of nourishment.

Can milk produce allergy?

Milk allergies include infantile eczema, asthma and gestro-intestinal allergy showing up as vomiting, diarrhoea and colic.

Cow's milk protein is the main cause of allergy.

Is there any relation between milk production and parity?

Provided mother is confident about her ability to breast feed there is no difference in quality of milk.

Is over breast feeding possible?

It is very difficult to over breast feed a child because he regulates his own supply. Over feeding generally takes place in bottle feeding and usually causes vomiting and diarrhoea. After a bottle feed the baby regurgitates a large amount of milk and passes large, stool several times a day. He also cries between feeds.

Is it possible to have pesticides in breast milk?

Theortically it is possible. Cow's milk also contains pesticides but as the formula milk is made of milk of many cow's from different areas, the amount of pesticides is reduced.

Is it possible to breast feed a premature baby?

Premature baby may be born before term or may be born at time but is small for date, i.e. below 2.5 kg. Both thrive better on breast milk. But low birth baby may require intensive baby care at nursery.

Can very low birth-weight babies be fed?

Babies below 1500 gm are unable to suckle at breast because their suckling and swallowing mechanisms have not developed well. Their digestive system is also not well developed to digest fat and sugar. Such babies may be fed intravenously or by tube.

Why do babies spit up after feeding?

Spitting up may be messy but don't worry. Infants often spit up after a feed in the first few months. The baby may trickle one or two mouthfuls of milk down his chin, onto your clothes while burping or taking a break from feeding.

(i) Avoid vigorous play and keep him upright for about ½ hour after he is finished.

(ii) Give him smaller feeds.

Are spitting and vomiting the same?

No, vomiting involves the forced expulsion of stomach contents with abdominal muscle contraction. Persistent vomiting needs attention because there may be an intestinal obstruction.

What the parents can do when a child vomits?

- Try to feed your baby before he is frantically hungry.
- Don't try to feed him when he is crying.
- Make feeding time calm and quiet.
- Burp the baby after each feed. Hold him upright.
- Avoid feeding while the child is lying down.
- If you are breast feeding your baby, feed 10-15 minutes on each side.
- Avoid interruptions, sudden noises, bright lights and other distractions.

Does the child spit up the whole of the feed?

When the child spits it seems that he has spitted out the total quantity. But it is not more than a table spoonful mixed with saliva and mucus. Usually it looks like curdled milk. It is messy and leaves stains on clothes. But it will not cause choking, coughing and discomfort. Don't allow the child to lie down on his stomach.

Why do children develop projectile vomiting?

In some male children vomiting begins between 2-4 weeks after birth. It may not develop after every feed. Condition is due to progressive narrowing of pylorus. Doctor should be consulted.

Sometimes the child refuses to feed, why?

The child may suck for a short time and then stop. Sometimes it may lead to distress in mother. Following suggestions may be useful.

- Make sure that the baby is comfortable and is able to breath comfortably.

- If your milk flow is fast, it may be choking the child.
- If your breasts are too full, express a little milk manually before feeding.
- Handle your baby calmly, gently and affectionately.

Can mother start breast feeding again after a gap?

A gap in breast feeding may happen due to many reasons –

- Child was kept away in hospital or so due to his illness.
- Mother misses the nurturing effect of breast feeding and is eager to resume.
- Child would have developed allergy to cow's milk.

It is not difficult to re-establish lactation but if the interval is a long one then it may be difficult. Although frequent suckling is the main point to re-establish breast feeding, to encourage the prolactin reflex mother can hand express the milk. Use of tablet metochlorpromide may help.

How does the excess salt in cow's milk affect the baby?

Cow's milk contains six times more phosphorus, four times more calcium and four times more sodium as compared to human milk. This may make the formula fed baby thirsty. Mother gives more of milk making child more thirsty.

What is the effect of smoking and breast feeding?

Cigarette smoking during pregnancy may result in abortion, increase the risk of hemorrhage and reduce birth weight. Certain studies show that smoking leads to disinclination to breast feed.

How child shows his willingness to take food?

Before 5 months a child cannot indicate to his mother that he does not want food and as a result he is over fed. After 5 months if he likes the food he may lean forward or open his mouth. If he had enough he will turn his head away.

Overfeeding with incorrectly mixed formula feeds and early addition of solid food may lead to obesity.

What kind of solid foods should be given?

Best is to start with mixed food. The food which the family eats, minced, mashed or strained. Home prepared baby foods are fresh and cheap. Marketed formulas may contain more of salt and sugar.

What precautions should be taken while preparing solid food at home?

- One should not overcook the food.
- Don't overboil vegetables. It will loose vitamins/minerals in water.
- Don't add salt or sugar which are unnecessary.
- Don't use canned fruits which may contain added salt and sugar.
- Don't force food to the child.
- Maintain high standard of hygiene.

What type of stools do breast fed babies have?

Stools of breast fed babies are often unformed, soft, mustard yellow in colour. Frequency of motion may vary. Breast fed babies may not pass stool for 3-4 days which is normal. When the baby opens his bowels the stool may be large.

Does breast feeding cause stretch marks on breasts?

Stretch marks on breasts, abdomen or thighs are caused by local damage to the lower layers of skin. It has nothing to do with breast feeding.

Can mother feed her twins?

Most mothers can feed them because the breasts automatically supply the extra quantity of milk needed. Many mothers may feed them simultaneously. Twins are often born before term and if baby is not fit to feed one can express breast milk and can give to the children.

What should be done if the baby is constipated?

True constipation in babies is rare. In constipation stool passed are small and hard like peanuts and while passing child may feel discomfort. To avoid it baby should be fed only on demand. Avoid forcing extra feed on him. Constipation may be relieved by adding a little sugar to the feed.

What do you understand by burping?

Every baby swallows some air during feed. If milk flow is slow more air is swallowed. Some of air comes up as a burp and rest passes down in intestine. This air emerges out with a noise.

What do you understand by posture feeding?

It is to feed lying down with your baby on top of you. It is comfortable. Most mothers find they need to posture feed for the early morning feed while in some cases she finds it necessary for her baby to finish the feed in the normal position to empty her breasts.

Can a mother who has undergone caesarean section breast feed her child?

A mother whose baby is born by caesarean section can breast feed. She has to be assured and encouraged. Because of operation she may have to try several positions to find a suitable position to feed.

Can breast and bottle feed both go together?

If mother is working or is not able to produce enough milk to satisfy her baby she may want to go on with a combination of breast and bottle feed. Both can be given together.

Should one avoid bottle feed in bed?

Yes, because it may cause dental caries specially when they fall asleep with milk in their mouth. It may also lead to ear infection. Some milk can come down to Eustachian tube and bacteria can grow in milk behind the eardrum causing infection.

How can the feeding at night be made comfortable?

There are many options

(i) Keep warm water in sterilized flask in bed room and whenever needed prepare the feed.

(ii) Keep the prepared food ready and warm it by putting the bottle in luke warm water.

(iii) Feed should never be kept warm in flask to feed during night because germs can breed.

> Knowledge helps you make a living; wisdom helps you make a life.

Weaning

Dr. Sujata

What do you understand by weaning?

It is the process of shifting from milk feed to semisolid food. If this change is made happily with baby's full interest then in future there will be no problem in developing his future eating habits. Undue fussing by mother can result in a lifelong food faddism or phobia.

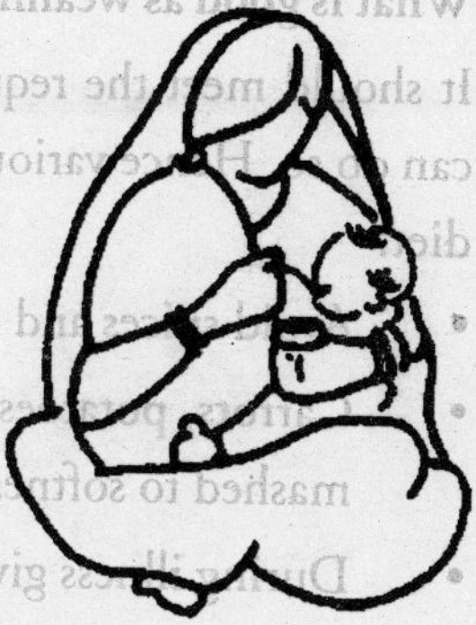

What should be the age to introduce semisolid food?

Breast milk provides sufficient food till 6 months of age. From the 6th month complementary food should be given for adequate growth. It will prevent malnutrition also.

6-12 months is the correct age when the child must be fed soft foods frequently and patiently. These foods should be given along with milk and not totally replacing milk. Breast feed may be continued for one year. If child is kept purely on milk then he may develop milk anemia which will lead to poor growth.

Why only after six months?

By six months an infant can voluntarily control sucking. He can swallow also. Hence he will not push out solids. In some cases teeth start erupting and pancreatic enzymes reach upto such levels that it can digest starch. By the age of 9 months an infant can clear a spoon. He can move food with the help of tongue. Solids can also be chewed.

What type of complementary foods can be given?

Suji and banana being soft are very suitable foods. The banana can be mashed. Consistency of food should be smooth. Some children may like liquid supplements. Such children can be started on semisolids and may then be given solids. Vegetable fibres may cause indigestion.

What is good as weaning food?

It should meet the requirement of the child but no single food can do so. Hence various types of food should be included in the diet.

- Avoid spices and chillies.
- Carrots, potatoes can be easily cooked along with dal and mashed to softness.
- During illness give small frequent meals.
- Fresh food may be mashed.

How frequently can foods be given?

mall amounts should be given two to three times a day. Gradually the amount of food may be increased. It is advisable to continue breast feed.

What should be the feeding practice at the age of one?

although the child can feed himself by the age of one year but he still needs supervision and help.

- Child should not be forced to have food.
- He should be introduced to one food at a time.
- Variety should be introduced in his diet. Colour, flavour and texture should be given due respect.

What points should be kept in mind by parents about food?

- They should provide a variety of health foods.
- Nuts, grapes and ground candies should not be given to infants because these can choke the child.
- Let the child decide how much he wants to eat.
- Food should neither be given as reward nor should the child be denied food as a punishment.

Can a baby bite the nipple?

Once the baby develops teeth he can bite the nipple. It happens because his gums tingle during teething. It becomes painful and nipples may become sore. But baby can be politely asked not to bite.

How soon should milk be used after been taken out of the refrigerator?

At room temperature bacteria can multiply rapidly. If more than 2 hours have lapsed since the milk had been taken out of the refrigerator and has been left in a room or a car, one should not use it. One should not use formula milk which is not cold to touch.

What are concentrated liquid formulas?

It generally comes in cans and has to be diluted in equal volume of water. Water should be sterilized. Pour the diluted formula into sterilized bottle and use immediately.

How to prepare powdered formula?

Generally ½ kg tins with measuring spoons and reclosable plastic lids are available of different companies. This is easier to carry while travelling. This needs to be mixed with distilled or boiled water. Powder and water has to be mixed properly avoiding lumps.

What are cow's milk formula?

In this type of formula butter fat has been replaced by vegetable oils. Carbohydrate, vitamins and minerals have been added. Protein content is reduced to suit the baby. In some cases, iron too is added.

Can an ill child be breast fed?

Why not. Breast feed has to be continued. If he is not able to suck strongly, frequent feeds should be given.

Can breasts produce sufficient milk to twins?

Yes, most of the mothers have sufficient milk to feed twins but will need a lot of support. Some are able to feed both babies at a time on different breasts while some feed one by one.

Should low birth babies be kept on breast feed?

- If the baby is too small and cannot suck, the mothers milk should be expressed on many occasions a day and expressed milk may be given to a child.
- Baby may be allowed to suck as often and as early as he can.
- Baby may be helped to put nipple in his mouth.
- Weigh the baby regularly to make sure that he is gaining weight.

What about HIV and breast feeding?

This is a complicated issue.

- Best way may be to avoid breast feeding.
- There is a 15% extra risk of mother to infant transmission.
- Counselling of HIV positive mother should be started from antenatal period.

- Anti retroviral treatment is a strategy for prevention of mother to child transmission of HIV.

What is the nutritional component of breast milk?

Breast milk is lower in protein than cow's milk. Milk contains two types of proteins and an insoluble protein casein which gives white colour. Human milk contains 60% whey. Cysteine content is twice that of cow's milk. Taurine needed for retinal development is present in a higher amount.

What about the fat in breast milk?

98% is triglyceride. This milk has a higher proportion of unsaturated fatty acids. Long chain derivatives of essential fatty acids are important structural compoments of brain present in mother's milk. Fat and energy content rises during the course of a feed. Fore milk is diluted and hind milk has double the fat content.

What type of carbohydrate is present in breast milk?

Lactose is present in high concentration in human milk. It helps in production of gut flora to avoid gastroenteritis. It further helps in calcium absorption.

What growth factors and hormones are available in breast milk?

Many hormones and growth factors are found in the human milk like epidural growth factor, insulin like growth factor, corticosteroids, thyroxine and prostglandins.

What about iron content in mother's milk?

When a child has a weight of about 5 to 6 kg, i.e. double the birth weight, iron reserves of the body become very less. Iron deficiency may impair neurodevelopment and immunity. Hence the baby needs iron-rich weaning food and supplemental iron drops.

How can a working mother continue to breast feed?

In non-organized area mothers do not get much of maternity leave to feed the child at home. This may be the cause of cessation of breast feeding earlier. The baby may be breast fed in early hours before going to work or she can express her milk in a clean container which can be fed to him by a caretaker later on in the day. Expressed milk, in cold weather, can be kept for 8 hours.

What are the benefits of breast feeding to the mother?

- It promotes early uterine evolution due to oxytocin release.
- Obesity is less common amongst breast feeding mothers.
- It has a protective effect against cancer of breast and ovaries.

Which is a option for feeding a bottle or a cup?

Bottle feeding can be avoided because most women do not know the importance of clean sterile bottles. Baby can also learn to drink from a cup.

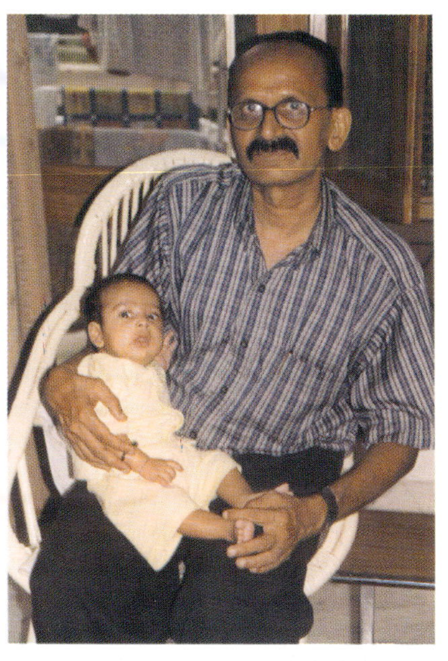

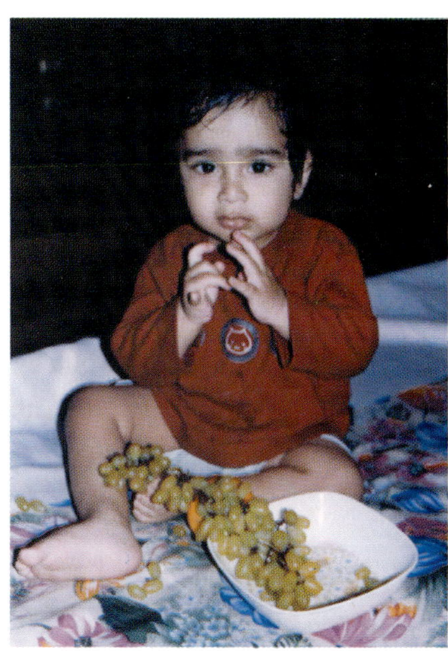

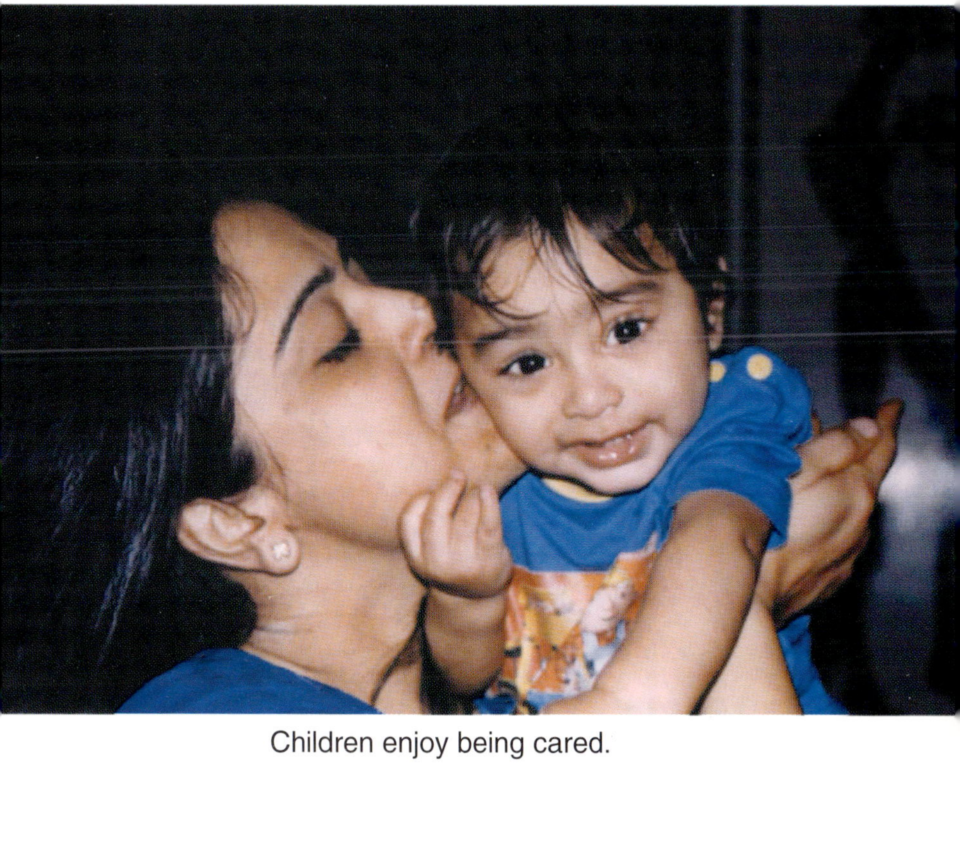

Children enjoy being cared.

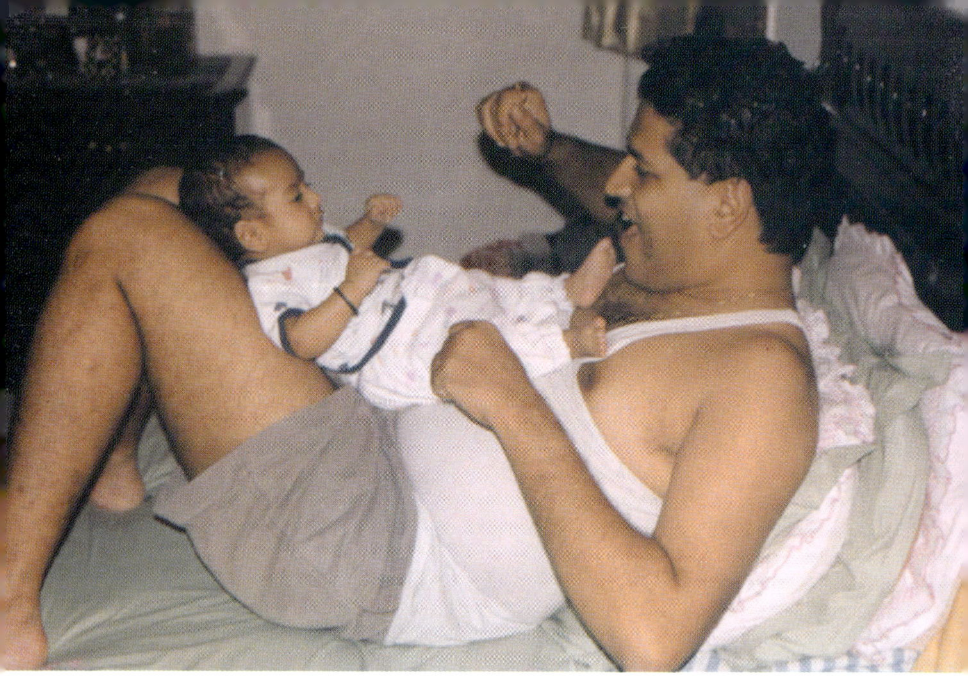

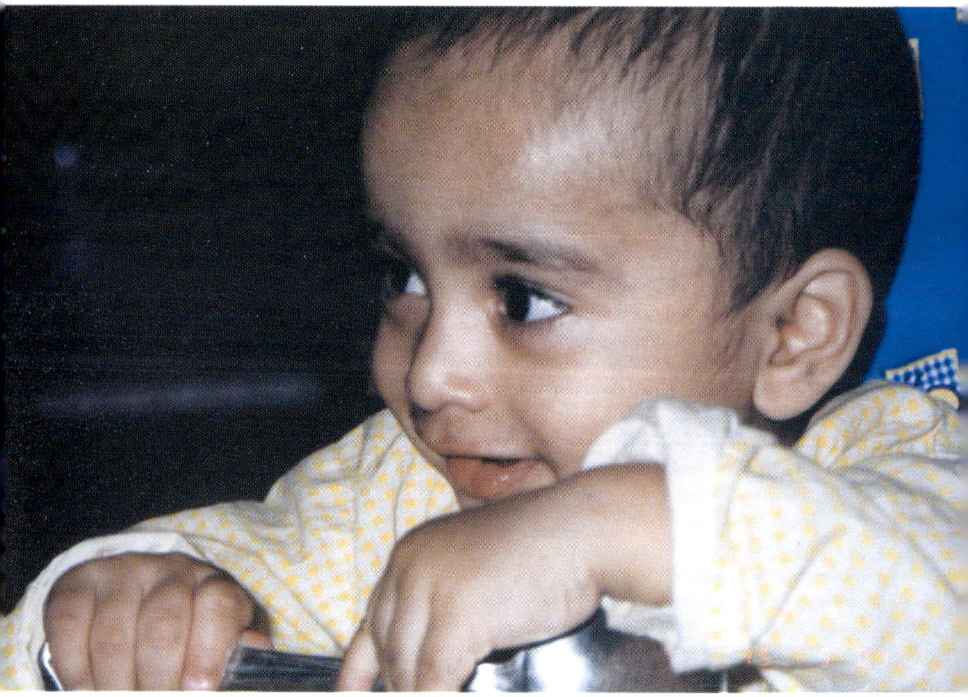

Naughty looks.

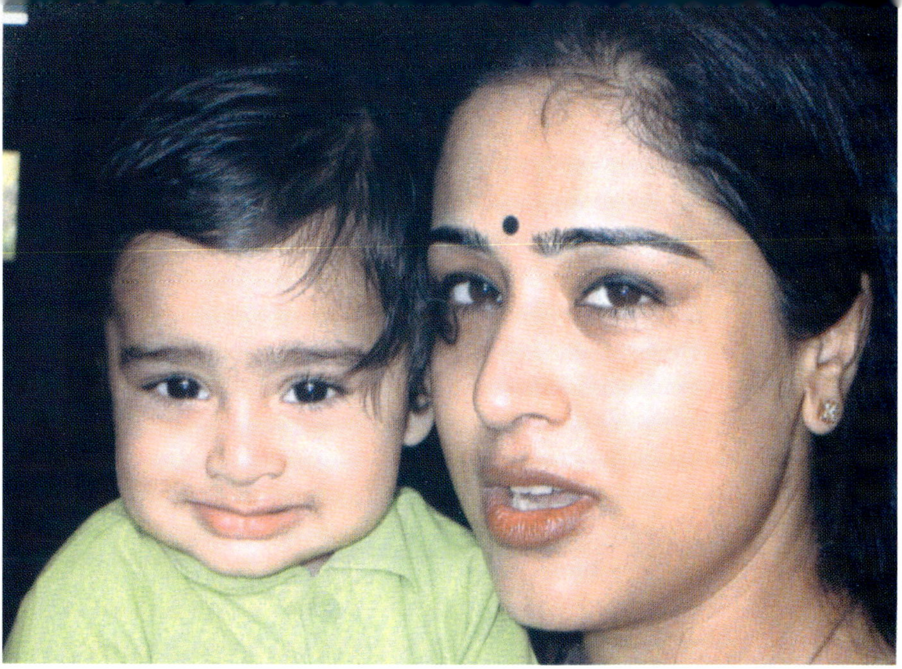

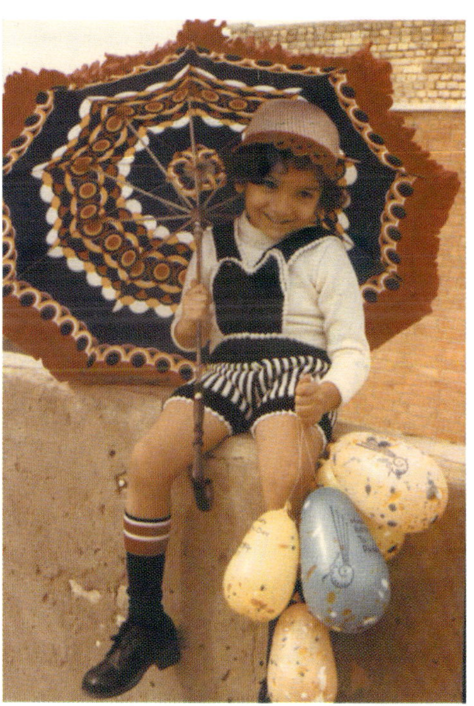

Mother & baloons are child's priorities.

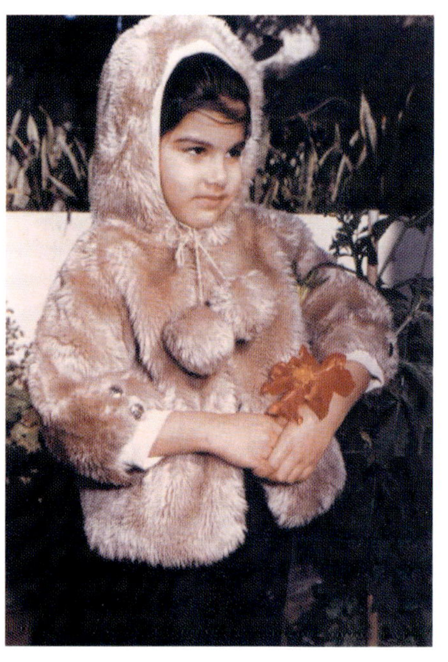

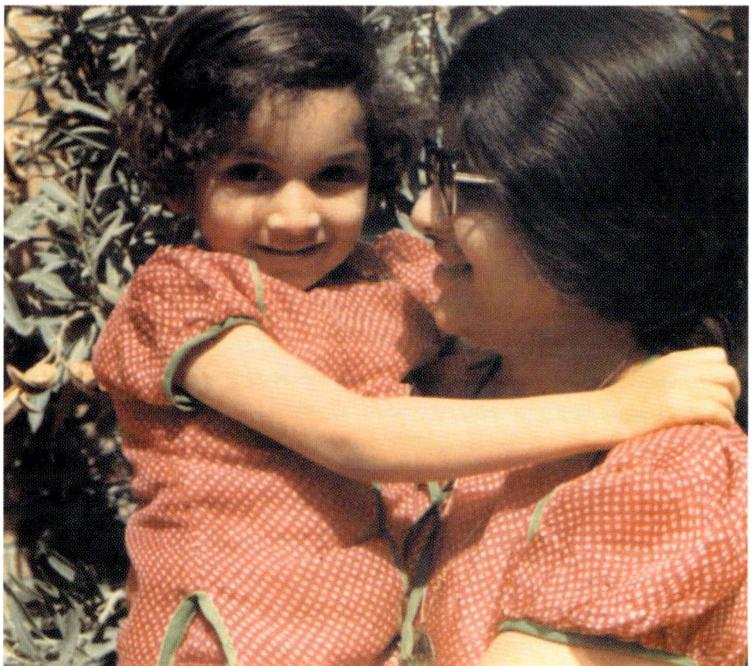

On occasion they prefer fancy dresses.

Growth and Development of Children

Jayshree Sahu, Kusum Gupta, Priyam Kotwal

From conception to adulthood there are periods of rapid growth and slow growth. Each child is different so there is no need to worry. Children born before time need extra care.

MILE STONES

What do you expect from a child of 1 month?

- He will raise his head if lying on tummy.
- He will be able to move arms and legs at one time.
- He will move suddenly on sharp noises.
- When close to you he will be able to watch your face.

How will a child behave at the age of 2 months?

- He will smile when he is spoken to.
- May turn head from side to side.
- Watches movements of others.
- Coos.

How does a child of 3 months behave?

- He will hold his head up.
- He can lift his head and chest when lying on his tummy.
- He can hold his hands together.

How does a child of 4 months react?

- He can roll back to his tummy.
- He can follow a person by moving his eyes.

- He can grasp objects.
- He can turn his head towards eyes.

What can a child of 5 months do?

- He can stretch his arms to be picked up.
- Knows familiar faces as well as sounds/voices.
- He may cry and make sounds to attract attention.
- He can reach for objects.

What are the milestones at the age of 6 months?

- He can raise his hands above his body.
- Sits with proper support.
- Rolls over.
- Begins finger feeding.
- Babbles and laugh.
- Tries to copy sounds.

What can a child of 7 months do?

- Moves object from one hand to other.
- He recognises and smiles at images in the mirror.
- Knows his parents.
- Appreciates his care givers.

How does a child of 8 months behave?

- He can sit alone.
- Can stand for a short period.
- Can creep.

What can a child of a 9 months do?

- He can crawl on his hands and knees.
- Picks up objects.

- Makes two sounds 'ga ga' and 'ba-ba'.
- Responds on being called by his name.
- May not like strangers.

What will be the development at 10 months?

- He understands 'no' and 'bye bye'.
- Looks out for hidden things.
- Hits together two objects held in his hands.

What is the progress at 11 months?

- Says 'ma-ma' or 'da-da'.
- Stands alone for a short period.
- Waves for 'good bye'.

How will a child of 12 months behave?

- He will comfortably say 'ma-ma' and 'da-da'.
- He can stand alone.
- He can walk with support.
- Self feeding with spoon starts.
- Copies others.
- He feels and understands commands.

How does a child of 15 months behave?

- Can speak 5 to 15 single words.
- He can give and take toys.
- He can walk well.
- He helps in dressing/undressing himself.
- He can drink from a cup hold in both hands.
- He listens to stories.

What does a child do at 18 months?

- He can walk up the stairs with help.
- Eats with spoon and fork.
- He likes to play with other children.
- He can point out the body parts.

How does a child of 2 years behave?

- He runs, jumps and throws ball.
- He can put on some clothes by himself.
- He can wash with hand.
- He can speak about 50 words.
- He can use 2-3 words at a time.
- He can open a door.
- He can tell his name if asked.
- Begins toilet training.
- He can find out where objects were kept.

How does a child of 3 years behave?

- He kicks ball.
- He can walk up stairs.
- Uses 3-4 word sentences.
- He knows his full name/sex.
- Dresses self but cannot button the shirt/pant.

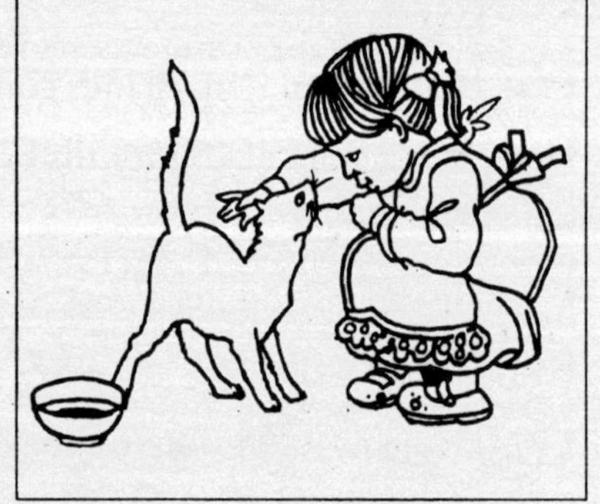

- Toilet training continues.
- He likes to play in small group with cats/dogs.

How does a child behave at the age of 4 years?

- He can catch a ball.

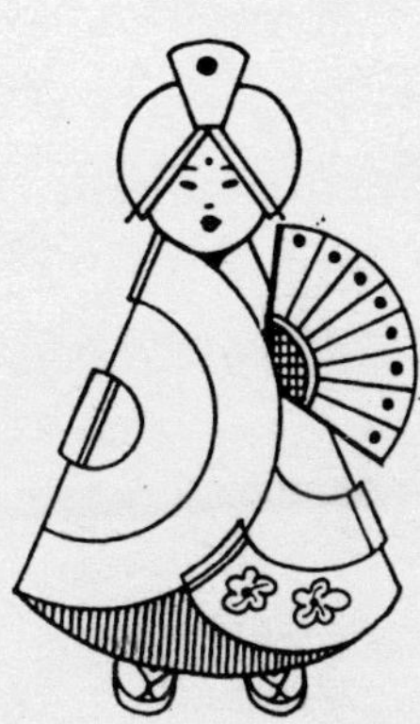

- Hops and stands on one foot.
- Washes hand comfortably.
- He can brush his teeth.
- He becomes well trained as far as toilet habits are concerned.
- He can share things.
- He can wait for his turn.
- He likes to have fancy dresses.

How will a 5 year old behave?

- He can tell a simple story.
- He listens and follows simple orders.
- He can count up to 100.
- He recognises colours.
- He can try to hit ball.
- He remembers some tables
- He can repeat rhymes.

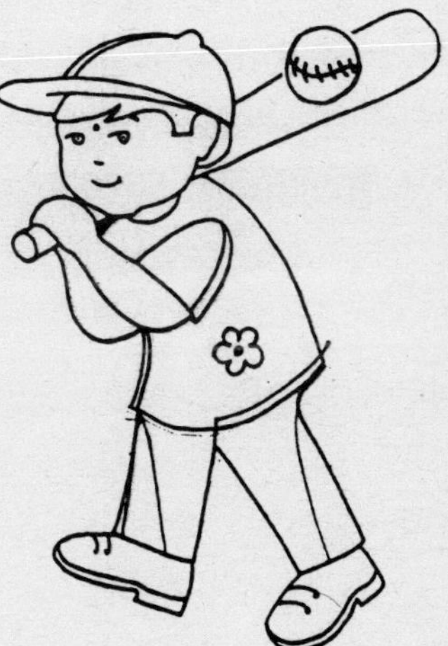

How does a child behave at the age of 4 years?

- He can catch a ball.

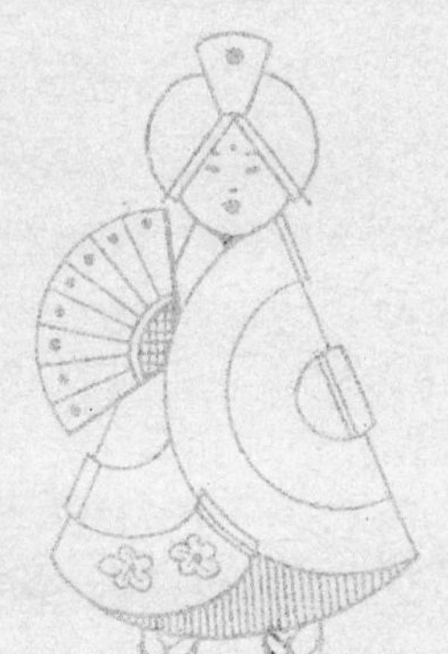

- Hops and stands on one foot.
- Washes hand comfortably.
- He can brush his teeth.
- He becomes well trained as far as toilet habits are concerned.
- He can share things.
- He can wait for his turn.
- He likes to have fancy dresses.

How will a 5 year old behave?

- He can tell a simple story.
- He listens and follows simple orders.
- He can count up to 100.
- He recognises colours.
- He can try to hit ball.
- He remembers some tables
- He can repeat rhymes.

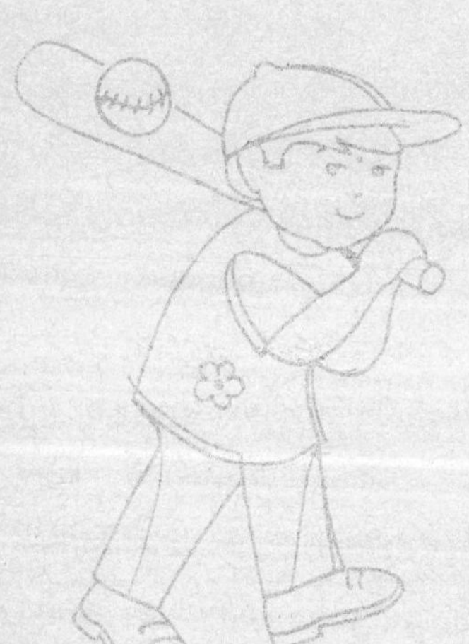

Social and Emotional Development

Dr. L. C. Gupta

How will a child reacts at the age of 1 month?

- His whole world is bounded by himself.
- He is concerned about his own needs and their satisfaction.
- He will start crying when he is hungry, or feels cold and hot.
- Little penetrates his mind.
- When he is satisfied he will not cry.
- If you talk to him when he is crying he may stop for a moment.
- He may make odd grimaces.
- He does not smile but seems to be doing so.

How is a child placed emotionally at the age of 3 months?

- He will kick quite vigorously when lying on his back. He can use both legs simultaneously or alternatively.
- One of his favourate activity is to play with his own hands, holding them up before his face and watching his fingers.
- He starts recognising his mother and follows her with his eyes.
- He does not like loud noises.
- He starts 'cooing' and gurgling.
- He is beginning to be a little more aware.
- He becomes very responsive to being touched or cuddled. He may enjoy gentle tickling.
- He is now sleeping less.

What is the emotional development at 6 months?

- He will scream with an annoyed sound in his voice to attract attention.
- He is much more aware of difference between himself and others.
- He becomes more aware of his own body.
- He plays with his fingers and toes as well.
- Generally he will use both hands to pick up things.
- He wants to put everything in his mouth. He uses his mouth to explore everything.
- He tries to hold a spoon.
- He is reaching the mimicry stage.
- He will be able to express his likes and dislikes through food.

What changes occur by the age of 10 months?

- He can turn his whole body to look sideways. He can stretch out to pick up something from floor.
- He can now be mobile. He can crawl on all four limbs throughout the room.
- He knows who he is and who are the people around him.
- He knows his mother well. He will start knowing his father and sibling. He will try to communicate with them by making vocal noises.
- He shouts to get someone to talk to him.
- He understands other people's communications.
- He will put his hand round his bottle or cup when feeding and try to get hold of the spoon when he is spoon fed.

- He may not like strangers and might hang on to known people.
- One of his favourite games is to drop spoon, food, toy and wait for the caretaker to pick it up.
- Another game he likes is putting things in and out of containers.

What are the emotional changes at the age of 12 months?

- He can stand and sit down without falling. He can stand for a shortwhile.
- He knows his name and responds on being called upon.
- He will like to go out of door for a stroll or a walk.
- His memory is developing and he can now find out his lost toy.
- He will know how to kiss and cuddle and enjoy doing it again and again.
- He likes to look at himself in the mirror. A child with a secure loving temperatment is one who has a loving and secure home.

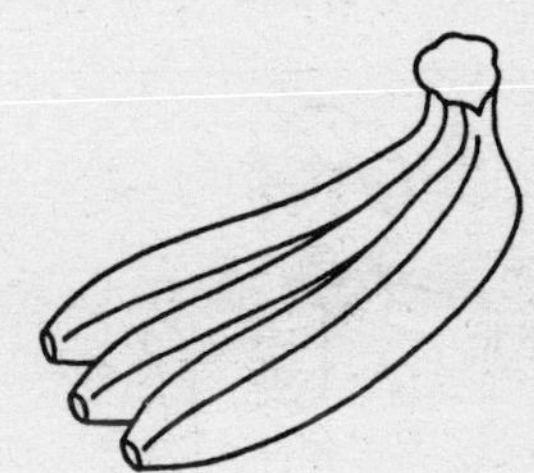

- He likes fruits, banana etc.

What is the emotional development at the age of 15 months?

- He may be able to bend over to pick things off the floor without tumbling.
- He can crawl up the staircase but find it very difficult to crawl down. The mother has to teach him to crawl down safely.
- He becomes more adventurous.

- He becomes fond of taking his clothes off, especially his shoes and socks.
- He becomes aware of his own bladder and bowel function.

How does a child react at the age of 18 months?

- By now the toddler can walk with his legs slightly apart.
- He can climb and descend the stairs.
- He can sit down in a chair by himself. He can run and jump rapidly.
- He shows more and more interest in books, pictures and sounds.
- He can point out what he wants.
- He enjoys rhythmic nursery rhymes and may try to sing.
- He can tell his mother when he wants to go to the toilet.
- This age is of negativism which means that whatever child is asked to do his answer is 'No'.

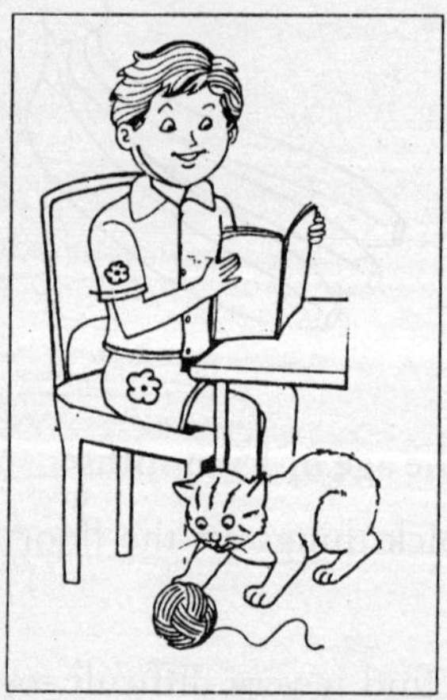

Love of a mother and her child is like the fusion of two chemicals. If there is any reaction both are transformed.

How will a child behave at the age of 2 years?

- He develops a definite personality. The personality can be accessed by his temperament whether he is restless or demanding, whether he is a highly intelligent child or an average one.
- If given paper and pencil, he will try to draw some circles.
- He is learning to recognise people face in photographs. He enjoys looking at photographs of members of his family.
- He can make believe and initiate to a marked degree.
- He is learning to play with other children.

What about general emotional development?

Some children are outgoing and extremely responsive to external events. These children require extra attention because they cannot tolerate any frustration. Such a child may well grow up to be a restless and ambitious person and a high achiever.

While on the other hand some children may not need much attention. They are easier to bring up. They are very happy to be by themselves.

Are all children equally loved?

Many children don't get sufficient mother's love because their mothers themselves did not get the desired love in their childhood. But a child could be cared for by someone who is his adopted parent, house servant/caretaker or any other substitute and still get enough love thus developing an emotional response. The person he loves is the one who cares for him.

However love grows and whoever gives it, what is important is the way it is expressed. There is no need to prove 'love'.

If a mother is distressed, depressed or frightened then her baby will often react by being miserable, crying a lot, feeding poorly or sleeping fitfully. If the mother is happy and contented the child will be happier.

Does a child need security?

A child who is loved as he needs to be has the first vital ingredient of security. It is a sense of being cared for. The ready availability of a mother is like having strong walls protecting him. Then only can he develop perfectly.

Sleep of A Baby

Dr. L. C. Gupta

Babies spend lot of time in sleeping.

A baby does not sleep for a long stretch at a time although he sleeps for about 16 hours.

Is sleep necessary?

Sleep is important for physical recuperation, immune system, physical growth, brain development, memory, learning and information processing. It is important as the baby is going through a difficult time adjusting to this world outside the womb.

How much sleep is necessary for a child of 3 months?

One should place the baby in crib when he is drowsy. If he is crying try to rock and cuddle him. Very young babies need to be held regularly otherwise they will cry. Light music may have soothing effect. During the day a baby may sleep for 3 hours at a stretch.

As baby grows older he will learn to sleep for longer hours.

What is the 'inverse rhythm of sleep'?

Some babies tend to sleep throughout the day and stay up all night. Such children have to be taken out of this hadn't. This could include more talking, playing, music etc during the day to keep him awake.

What is the sleep pattern at 3 months?

It is a good idea to have the crib of the child in a different room separate from the parents. Parents will not be able to respond to every cry and coo, and this way the child will know that it is a sleep time.

What will be the sleep pattern at 6 months?

Now four to five partial awakening at night are likely to be common.

How will a child sleep at 12 months?

At this stage children are aware and curious. Some may even fight their sleep. Try for a regular schedule. Day time crankiness will result in troubled nights.

Your baby's sleeping area should be dimly lit. Train your baby to associate a particular place with going to sleep even when it comes to a nap. As your baby gets older he will learn through association. Every night if you change him in to his night suit and shut off the lights, he will come to know that it is the time to go to sleep.

Is bed time a good opportunity to develop bonding?

It is a nice chance for parents to spend some time talking to their baby. Singing a lullaby is a time-tested way to help a sleepy baby drift off.

Safe Home and Equipment

Kusum Gupta

Why safety of home is necessary?

A woman carrying a child has to walk carefully. Floors should not be rough nor should it be slippery. Floors should be of non slip surfaces. Stairs should be covered by carpets if it can be afforded. Stairs with open risers are not recommended. Small children can slip through or may trap their heads in between them. Windows require special care and should never be easily openable.

Doorknobs should be at a height. Doors of the bathroom or kitchen should have a high set up of knobs. Bolts or keys should never be accessible to children because they may lock themselves in a room and lose the keys.

What should be the room temperature?

There can be 'neonatal cold injury' if a child is nursed below 65^0F. This develops because he does not have an inbuilt thermostat system – a muscle activity which burns up more fuel and thereby increases the body temperature.

What are the symptoms of cold injury?

The baby looks perfectly well or even rosy. But he is lethargic and may not like to feed. On touch he will be cold.

In order to avoid this, the room temperature should be between 65^0 and 70^0F.

What type of electrical equipment should be there?

All electric wires should be well protected and properly sealed. Fittings should not be loosely done.

What type of bedding should be used?

Smooth cotton sheets are good for summers. Blankets should be light, warm and easy to wash. Babies don't need pillows at all during the early months and will start using one only after the age of 2 years. Even if the mother wants to provide pillows, they must be of porous material such as foam rubber.

What type of clothes will a child need?

Nylon and terylene wash well and dry very quickly and don't need ironing but are less porous and therefore less comfortable. In India cotton, although difficult to maintain, suits well.

What type of nappies are best suited?

Fabric nappies laundered at home may be used. Secondly there are disposable nappies available in the market which require no washing at all and are virtually sterile. But these are costlier.

Is it necessary to sterilize fabric napkins?

Yes, it is necessary to sterilize fabric napkins, because if they are not free of germs and if the child wets it, the germs will grow faster. A nappy smells strongly not because of urine but because of bacterial action if the nappy is wet.

How to sterilize napkins?

Best way is to use a chemical such as hypochlorite. It safely sterilizes and softens nappies. Boiling can be effective but it requires twenty minutes of hard boiling. Napkins should be fully dipped in water. Boiling of nappies in hard boiled water may make nappies rough which may damage the baby's skin.

What type of prams are useful?

There are some very attractive small size prams now available which take up minimum of space and are easily dismentlable for storage. But a pram should be large enough to carry a large toddler. It's brakes should be safe and effective.

> Don't riducule children, their appearance, looks and personal traits. They will be become rebellious.

Play and Toys

Kusum Gupta

Play is the first work any of us do. In childhood playing is a source of information. It is as essential for normal development as food, drink and mothering.

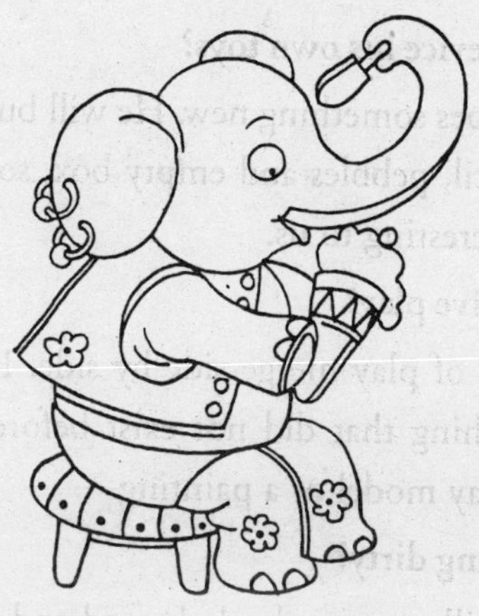

What is the purpose of play?

It provides sensuous satisfaction when a child starts breast feed. Breasts are also a toy for him. While playing with breasts he comes to know that fingers are sensitive, that lips are very sensitive and the tongue is even more. When he sucks his own thumb or toe he is exploring his own body. A child can absorb the available information so rapidly that very soon he feels tired and needs another set of toys.

Does a child like coloured toys more?

Yes, for closer vision a set of coloured balls, bells and rattles can be strung over the cot or pram. These may be within the vision of sight and reach.

What is the importance of imitative play?

It is the play through which a child learns the skill of being a person. He immitates sounds and out of this develops speech. He learns to close and open the eyes. As he grows older he immitates every thing. Being very close to the mother he will immitate mother's action.

Can a child device his own toys?

Every child does something new. He will busy himself with even a pen or pencil, pebbles and empty box, something which may be not be interesting to us.

What is creative play?

Various types of play merge side by side. In creative play child makes something that did not exist before. It may be a brick building, a clay model or a painting.

What is playing dirty?

Child may spill water and splash sand and mud. Such a child is really a creative person. Such play is necessary. A child can release anger, anxiety and confusion this way.

What denotes 'destructive play'?

Much of human creative work has to be preceded by destruction. The child who pulls a toy to pieces is actually not breaking it but he wants to know more about it.

How to choose a toy?

Following points should be kept in mind.

- Is the toy rich in play potential?
- Is the toy strong and will it stand to rough handling?
- Decide whether you are purchasing a toy for the child or simply because you have liked the toy.
- Is the toy educative to child or not?

Which toys are unsuitable?

- Too many toys are little more than ornament only.
- Toy should not have rough edges.
- Detachable small pieces may be swallowed by the child.

What are the toys for specific age group?

- Birth to 6 months – Rings, crumpled papers, strings of large beads.
- 6 months to 1 year – Rocking horses, push and pull toys.
- 1-2 years – Building blocks. Shape matching. Jumping jacks.
- 2-5 years – Dolls, cooking equipment, doll's furniture. Lego blocks.
- 6-8 years – Calculating dolls. Toy cars and activity toys.

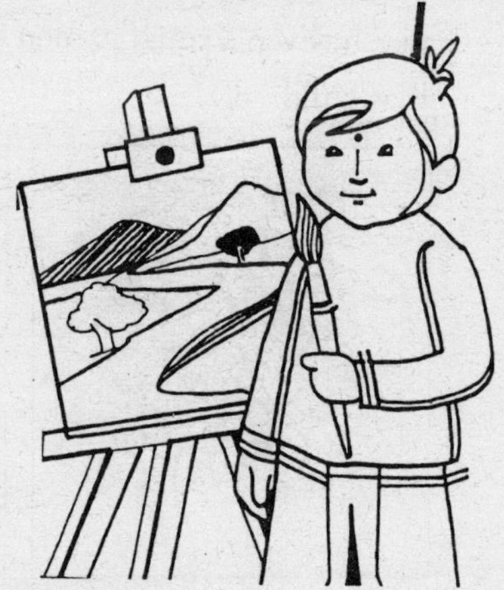

Which toys suit all ages?

Some toys are suitable for all ages, because requirement of different age groups overlap each other.

- Building bricks in natural colours.
- Construction toys.

- Jigsaw puzzles of different shapes.
- Painting equipment.

Do children like books?

- From the point of view of a child, books should have hard cover and be strong. He will try to tear it out.
- For an older child pages should be made up in such a way that the binding will hold them firmly. Book should be opened flat.
- Children like either very large or very small books.
- Books should have pictures of recognisable objects.
- Books should not have frightening pictures.

What about outdoor play?

Most of the children want to go out of the house with a grandparent for a walk. Even much smaller babies feel happy outside house. They see many moving objects of different shapes and colours. They see small pets and produce sounds of happiness.

A child feels happy playing with children of the same age group.

Do children like garden trees and multicoloured flowers?

Very much. Even a small garden can be made suitable for adults as well as children.

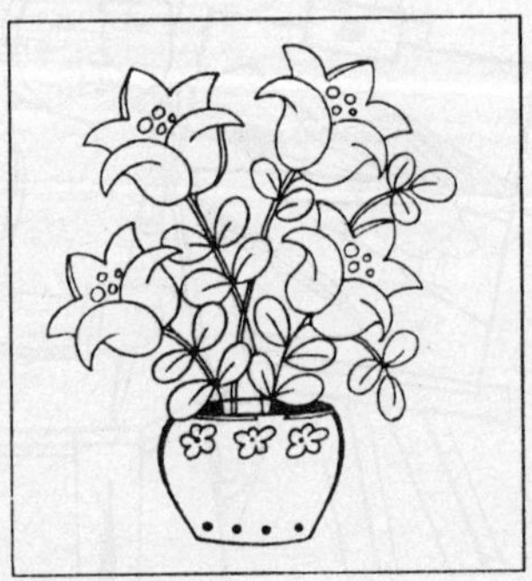

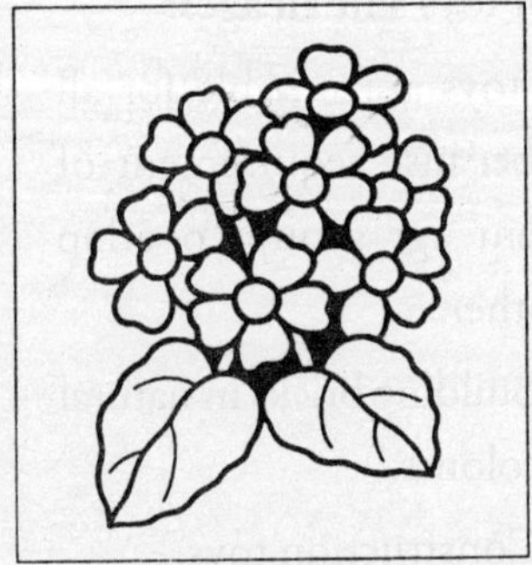

Play things for the garden can be made easily. Discarded car tyres can be hung from trees. Sand pits and slides are interesting for children. A garden should not have any poisnous plants.

It is better not to have a water pool in the garden. If there is one, then the water level should be very low. The pool should have fencing so that a child may not fall in it.

Inflatable pools are also not safe becuase they puncture very soon.

Do children like to visit zoos?

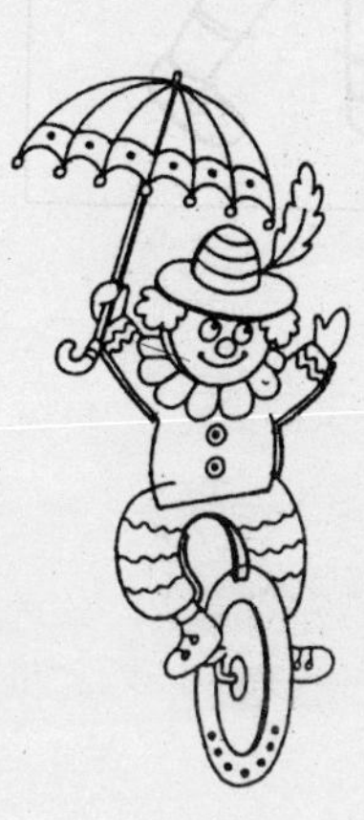

Yes very much. They get deeply interested in seeing deers, tigers, elephants, etc. Even infants gets excited and produce gurgling sounds.

Visiting a circus is great fun to them and the joker attracts them the most.

Do male children want to play with dolls?

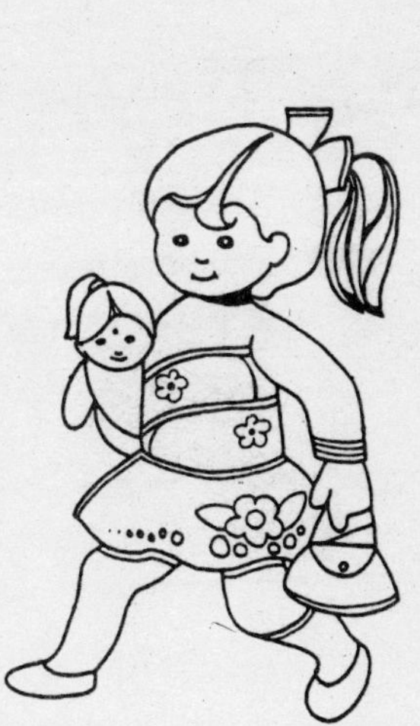

Traditionally no, playing with dolls and kitchen items is a passion for girls while boys like power games and toys like guns etc.

Do children like to play competitive games?

Yes, older children develop the feelings of competition. Even girls like to play ball, may be without net and goal.

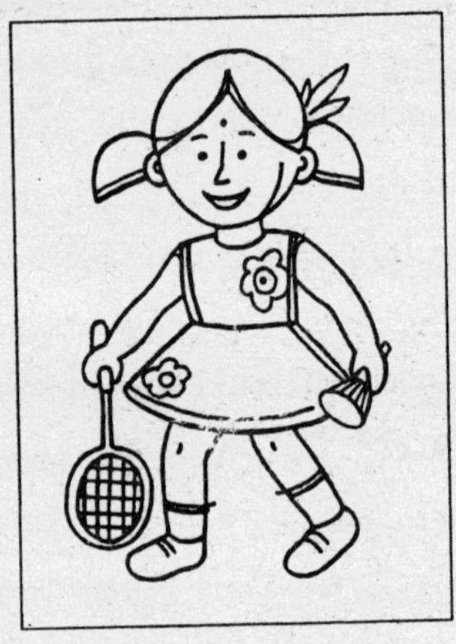

Discipline of Child

Dr. L. C. Gupta

'Discipline' sorely perplexes parents. They don't know when a child is expected to be obedient, what sort of punishment is needed and when.

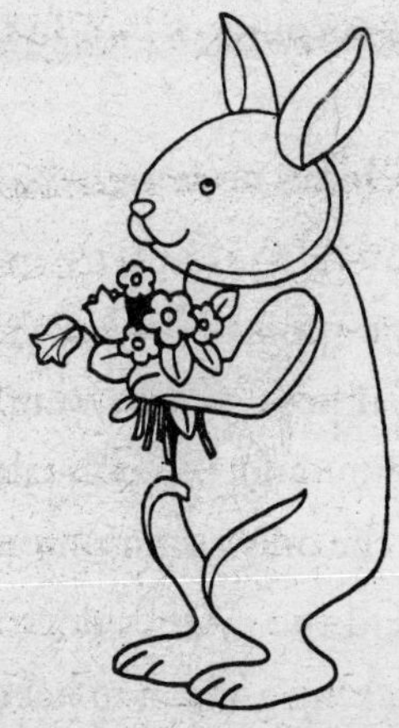

What is self-discipline?

Discipline needs to be directed towards helping the child to develop self-discipline. If his parents are harsh then the child will learn less. But if he is told why he should not do something and is helped to control and guide his own feelings then he will develop strength of character himself.

When are the roots of good discipline laid?

It is during the early months that the roots of good social behaviour are laid down. Most of babies are selfish and they only bother about their own needs. A grown-up with a baby's selfishness is a very unhappy person indeed and is known as 'spoiled'.

Who is a spoiled child?

A spoiled child is one who demands his own way constantly. He keeps everyone dancing on his tune. But a spoiled child is an unhappy one. Although his mother tries to satisfy him, his demands are never ending and he scowls more than he smiles. Actually speaking, a child's demands should not be met immediately because it encourages him to feel that he is right to cry for what he wants.

What can happen if a child's need are not met immediately?

On the other hand if a child's needs are not met promptly, it is possible that he may be spoiled by this rigidity. Think, if he is hungry he wants food, if he is cold he wants warmth and if he is lonely he needs company and the only alternative available to him is to cry. Crying is the only communication available to him.

If he keeps crying and the mother does not respond she may have false feeling of teaching a lesson to her child. In actuality she has taught him to despair. He still continues to have painful feelings plus a sense of total abandonment because he is not offered any relief. He learns that only if he screams for a long time then only anyone helps and if he does not scream he may be left alone – in return he is labelled as a spoiled child.

Does meeting needs of a child give a feeling of security to him?

If his mother comes with food and warmth and loving company, a child is helped to feel 'secure'. He comes to know that he is not alone and is cared for. As he grows he becomes a contented person.

What else does a satisfied child learn?

A satisfied infant learns to laugh and smiles a lot as a response to care and affection. A child's smile makes his mother more loving and more willing to be with child.

Can a grandmother discipline the child in a better way?

It is true that a grandmother has more experience to handle children effectively than the mother. It is perfectly normal for a child of a working mother to spend an afternoon cheerfully with his grandmother. Even then he waits eagerly for his mother to come from office.

At what age child may not need the mother's attention?

Desparate need for mother start slowly from the age of three. But everyone of us remembers our mother in times of stress. This probably comes from the feeling of deep attachment.

How to encourage the child to show good behaviour?

One good way is to offer him love. Mother may find some moments to go to the playing child and hug and kiss him and say 'I love you'. When this is done frequently child comes to equate good behaviour with maternal love.

Why does a child become naughty?

Naughtiness may be a demand for love. If the child behaves nicely the mother leaves him to play and become busy in other activity but if he becomes naughty she leaves those tasks and concentrates on him.

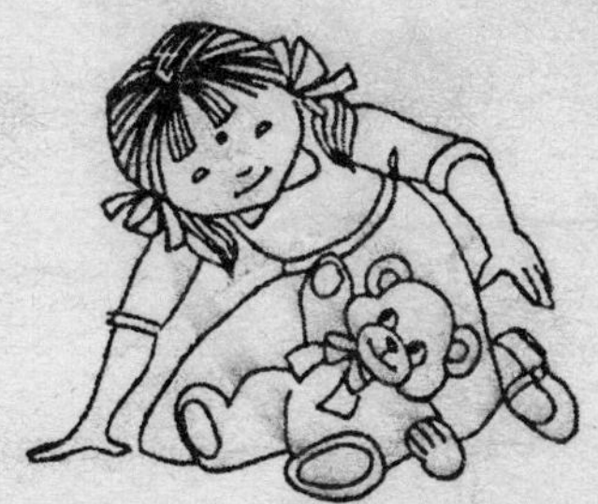

Should a child be given corporal punishment?

I am strongly not in favour of hitting

a small child. To me it is an admission of failure to understand the real needs of a child. With corporal punishment, the child will learn to lie and to avoid his parents and not to listen them.

Why do certain children become aggressive?

Some children hit out at other kids. They may hit even their own mother, destroy their property and toys of others. Even for such children corporal punishment is not the answer. It will only make them more aggressive. You must remember that aggressiveness is always a manifestation of insecurity and a demand for love.

What do you understand by temper tantrum?

Some children lie down on floor, kick and shriek, when prevented from doing what they want. Nothing will stop them except tiredness. One has to wait till the storm subsides, then reassure the child. Some children blackmail their parents this way and continue to have tantrums.

What is toddler rebellion?

From the age of a 1 to 3 or 4 the child seems to resist his mother at every turn. Whatever the mother wants him to do, his reply is 'No'. Rather he will do opposite. This is normal. A child who has never rebelled would never grow up in normal way.

Pre-school Child

Dr. Jad Aoun

Can a child develop well in any family?

Yes child can grow up with a healthy sense of respect and dignity in any sort of family, whether rich or poor. It depends on the parents' decision about what values will be taught to shape a child's life. A child can grow up healthy in any family built on love, respect and dignity.

What really happens in the name of love?

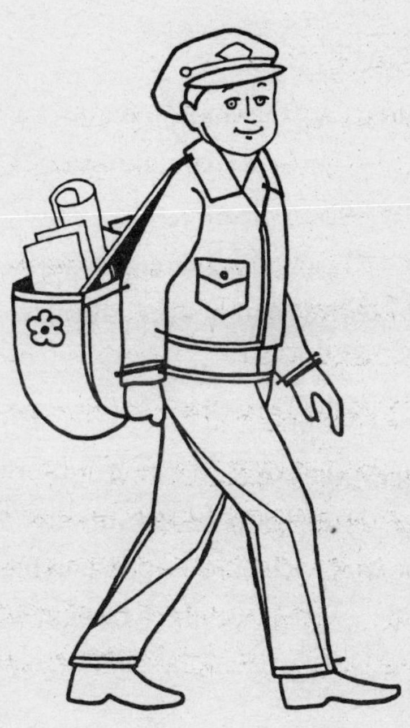

Every parent loves his or her child. But parents do many ineffective things in the name of 'love'. We should, however, love in ways that nurture accountability and self-esteem, encouraging children to reach their full potential as happy contributing members of society.

What significant change takes place in the second half of pre-school years?

Children begin to make relations with other people. A child finds friends. He notices skin colours, body shape and life style different than his own. He begins to make decisions which may lead to conflicts with his parents. Parents should learn to see the child as capable, able to master new skills and, in the process make mistakes.

What changes happen to a child at the age of 5 years?

A child now finds the most interesting children, his peer group. What the other children say, think and do register is vitally important. He feels that now he has not remained the centre of interest in family. At this age the seeds of empathy are planted. At this time parents should nurture co-operation.

What are the big changes a child notices while going to school?

The lunch box represents a concrete or visible change for a child. He gets a uniform and a pair of shoes. These special possessions provide him support.

Can 'Aya' look after a child, well?

Entrusting the care of a young child to another person requires a great deal of faith. It is very different to provide love to meet the needs of a child as parents naturally do.

When a mother goes away to work each day a farewell kiss is necessary. Holding a child before he waves from door is critical to emotional well being of parents.

How does a child communicate his feelings?

He may throw a toy across the room, fall over in a tantrum or collapse in a flood of tears and all within a span of a few minutes. It becomes difficult enough to cope with such emotions. A parent has to decipher his personal nonverbal clues. Learning to recognise and deal with a child's feelings is a vital step in handling children's behaviour.

What is a child's feeling?

Child learn to cope with his feelings by watching his parents. If parents deal with difficult feelings by fighting each other or by abusing, it leaves a damaging scar on the mind of the child. A temper tantrum is an emotional display.

Feelings are our scale, our way of keeping a watch over our activities.

How to teach children the difference between feelings and action?

Children need to learn that feelings are different than actions. One has to teach a child to deal with feelings and to express them in such a way so that they may not hurt him or others. A young child often chooses inappropriate ways to express his feelings, not because he is bad but because he is still learning to react.

Is eye to eye contact the best nonverbal communication?

Eye contact signals attention. It sends a message to the child that he is important, captures his attention and increases the effectiveness of our message. But unfortunately adults tends to make direct eye contact most often when an adult is angry or lecturing the child. In some cultures eye contact with elders is regarded as a sign of disrespect.

Is proper posture needed to make eye contact with child?

Yes, even if you want to communicate him, kneel next to him, sit beside him on sofa or set him on a counter where his eyes can meet yours comfortably.

How does the tone of voice affect communication?

Your tone of voice may be the powerful nonverbal tool. Your voice should be sweet and encouraging. Children are very sensitive to our nonverbal communications.

Can active listening be a effective tool of communication?

Yes, active listening is the art of observing and listening to feelings.

It does not mean that you agree with the child but it is an opportunity given to child to express himself. Active listening will help your child to learn about his own feelings.

What is the role of anger?

Tantrum is one typical expression of pre-school anger. Parents can help children begin to understand why they get angry, to know how that powerful emotion begins in their hearts and to develop ways that help them to cope and overcome anger.

When do they learn gender identity?

Children will learn to notice physical differences between boys and girls and often they will ask what it means. In these days of television/advertisement question may come even earlier. Little boys want to touch their fathers in the shower. Watching a mother feeding younger brother or sister may lead to all sorts of interesting questions. Parents should remain calm, relaxed and open to questions. Never scold the child for being inquisitive.

It is always wise to answer questions in simple accurate terms. With the help of books and pictures a child can be made to understand. Treat boys and girls with respect. Limiting children to gender specific roles will limit their capabilities.

When to tell a child that he is an 'adopted' child?

There is no clear answer to this. But too much information before the age six only confuses a child. But some believe that later a child is told, the more upsetting the news may be. Next question the child will ask his adoptive parents is who are his actual parents?

Parents should give many opportunities to experience belonging to the child so that he is aware of his worth and significance too.

Is it necessary to show affection, interest and acceptance?

It has been shown that children who receive warm, consistent loving care produce less of the stress hormone cortisol and even if they become upset, they become normal rapidly. On the other hand, children who suffered abuse or neglect in early life are likely to feel more stress frequently and with less provocation.

Should a parent practice the art of conversation?

Children develop language by speaking and by being spoken to. Conversation with pre-schoolers is an art requiring both humour and patience. You should not speak to young children in ways that don't allow for much response.

Will reading help the child?

It is never too soon to start reading books. Books open new worlds to children. Pictures stimulate thinking and learning. Babies like colourful pictures. They usually have their own favourite books and stories.

Should a child's curiosity be encouraged?

Pre-school is the time when a child is discovering himself and is eager to explore and experiment with his own interest and abilities.

Parents should provide lots of safe opportunities to run, climb, jump and explore. Honour your child's interests. These children want to do rather than just watch.

Should television time be restricted?

Television has become the centre of interest in many families. Excessive television may be actually changing the way the brain functions. Because it is a passive activity, one way traffic and conversation is not there. Children who see lot of television have more of weight problem and show less of creativity in their play.

Children do imitate what they see on the television, and this may even mean jumping from a height.

Do you need to teach discipline?

Best sort of discipline is teaching. Shame, punishment and humiliation will make a child shy and fearful. Positive discipline skills are encouraging for brain development.

Should one recognise and accept a child's uniqueness?

A child learns about himself and the world by watching and listening. What he decides about himself depends on what messages he receives from his parents and caregivers and he develops a sense of self-esteem on the basis of this.

What are the advantages of sending a child to a 'play school'?

Remember that success at school is more than academic skills. A child learns to tolerate time away from parents. He learns to respond to a teacher, make friends with other children. Children do better with academic learning.

What is the myth of a perfect child?

For most of the people a 'Perfect child' is often pictured as one who is sober, obeys parents, does not fight with others, who is keen of learning and is popular. But very few children fit into this fantasy description.

What should be the activity level?

Activity level refers to a child's level of motor activity and proportion of activity and inactivity periods. Plan ahead with your child's needs in mind. Provide him a space to run off excess energy. Take him to parks, or if possible and feasible enroll him in swimming classes. You should match your expectations to your child's capabilities.

What about the sensory threshold?

Some children wake up from a nap everytime a door opens no matter how softly, while others can sleep through disco music. The level of sensitivity varies from one child to the next.

What about the quality of mood?

Some children react to life with pleasure while others can find fault with everybody and every thing. So parents should be sensitive to their child's mood and should pet him off and on.

What is the intensity of reaction?

Every child responds to situations differently. Some react to a situation with action and emotion while others look and smile and go back to work.

Should parents behaviour be firm and kind with a child?

Parents should be kind but should handle the child with firmness. Kindness shows respect for the child and his uniqueness while firmness shows respect for the need of the situation.

Do children develop special friendships?

5 year old child is at the peak of being social and loves to play complicated games. Catastrophe threatens when one member of a special friend group links up with another, excluding the third. Being left out is painful. Special friendships form important foundations for many of life's relationships.

Why nobody likes a particular child?

A child who is hurting others or who refuses to co-operate in games is not liked by other mates. Parents should guide such children to be more adjustable and kind to others.

What is the advantage of a only child?

An only child is the recipient of his parents' undivided love and attention. He is highly motivated but being lonely may not develop the sense of adjustment and sacrifice. He becomes slow at learning to share.

What is the role of an eldest child?

Such a child often acquires language quickly and is the dear one of whole family. He has more privileges in the family but much is expected from him in return. The eldest one is always under pressure to do 'best', an example to juniors to be followed.

How does 'youngest child' enjoy life?

He is a member of a special class. For him rules are relaxed although other siblings may perceive the youngest one as a spoiled one. Such child gets most toys and stuff.

How does the middle child feel?

A middle child feels lost in the family. He depends on other siblings for support and encouragement. He does not get the privileges of either the oldest neither does he receive the special treatment of the youngest. He is treated unfairly and may become hostile in his effort to create a place of belonging.

What about quarrelling of pre-school children?

When such children are fighting their parents should ask them to sit quietly to cool off and calm down. Adults should not loose their own tempers.

What about hitting and aggression?

Children who are hitting or pulling hair should be firmly separated. It is to be understood that such behaviour often contains a coded feeling.

What happens when children hurt adults?

Sometimes pre-schoolers learn to hit, kick and bite their parents if life does not go their way.

There are many ways to deal with this. Leave the child alone or if you are worried that he will tear up clothes or hurt himself, try to hold him firmly so that he cannot kick. Rocking gently may calm him down.

What is to be done if child still misbehaves?

Even with the best training it is unrealistic to expect perfect behaviour. One day the child will start running after a forbidden object. Parents should keep expectations reasonable. Think your action thoroughly before threatening to child.

Why does child abuse take place?

All parents feel frustrated at one point of time. Some adults have never experienced loving, effective parenting themselves so do not know what to do. Child abuse in all forms, verbal, physical, emotional and sexual is a complex subject. Parents are under financial or emotional stress or have unrealistic expectations from their child.

Is parenting an act of courage?

The responsibility of raising and guiding a child needs courage. It increases as the child grows. When a child does not obey and refuses to eat, we all loose our courage. Fear and weariness take over and we become discouraged.

What if a child makes mistakes?

Actually we all make mistakes. This is normal and not always a sign of failure. We make mistakes, learn from them and move on.

Children need to be encouraged. Encourage the child to do what he can instead of what he cannot.

What about pre-school children and potty training?

Many children become potty trained before they reach the age of three. Any delay is this could be due to power struggle between the adult and the child.

Potty training is just a training. Involve your attitude. If you are relaxed and comfortable your child will also be relaxed. Pressure to 'succeed' will frustrate both of you. If your child is wet change him but you should never over humiliate your child for this.

Are there setbacks in potty training?

New location, new environment and travelling, all of these may cause training to suffer a setback. If parents' attitude is not co-operative child may also be confused.

What is the role of grandparents?

Many children spend their time with grandparents. In fact many grandparents are raising the children when the mother is a working lady. Under such circumstances the child may become more attached to the grandparents. The grandparents take the child for a walk, spend money on chocolate and ice creams. They carry the child to school and bring him back home. For such children 'Ba' means 'Baba' and 'Baba' means 'Bazar'. They simply want to go out of home with him.

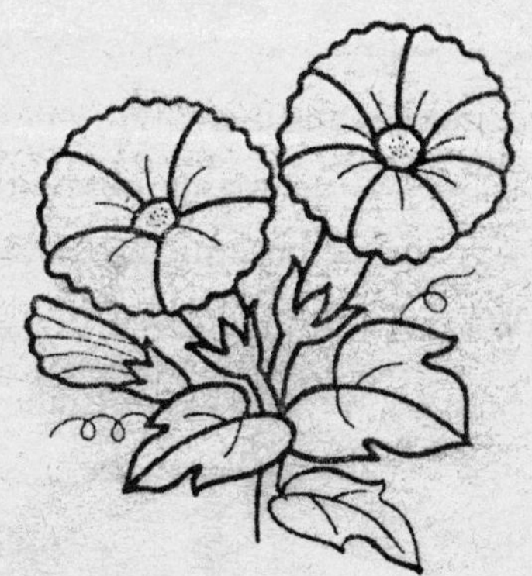

Anti-social Behaviour

Dr. A. K. Saxena

Between the ages of 2 to 5 a years wide range of behaviour patterns develop which alarms the parents. Actually it is very difficult to decide what is normal and what is not. Some behaviour may be anti-social.

What about a child's aggressiveness?

If we think seriously we will realise that aggressiveness is a true life force. It is a part of self-esteem, part of loving as well as hating. In some societies an aggressive nature in males is admired.

But what most people are concerned about is the attempt to show physical violence, shouting and screaming.

How to deal with a child's aggression?

It is very important not to treat boys and girls differently. But many parents tolerate aggressive behaviour in boys but not in girls. Aggressive behaviour is the outcome of anger, frustration and distress. So the best way is to prevent such experience. To punish the child is itself an aggressive behaviour on the part of the caretaker.

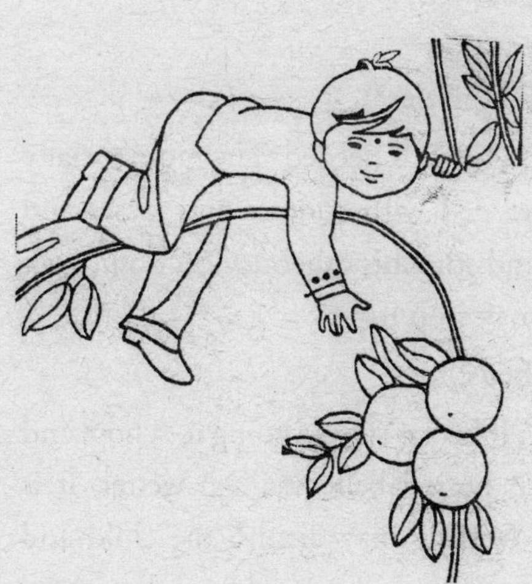

What is required is to teach the child to direct his aggression in a way that gives him relief without harming himself or others. One has to prevent physical aggression by holding him is one's arms. The child has to be held closely and lovingly. Then he gets the reassurance he needs and is better able to handle his own feelings.

From where does a child pick up the idea of aggressiveness?

The child picks up ideas from his surroundings very quickly. If parents are aggressive to each other then he too will be the same. A husband who hits his wife, cannot have a son who is a gentle and tender man.

If a child is aggressive without any reason and the problem continues, then consult the family doctor.

What are attention getting devices?

A child needs his mother's undivided attention. When a second child comes the first starts getting envious. How it starts is really irrelevant. What is needed is to recognise what the child wants and why he is making a fuss. One should satisfy him. Do not surrender like a doormat but give all the reassurance that you can give.

How to deal with a child who grizzles?

For a child who grizzles a firm tactis is needed. The more socially acceptable behaviour is rewarded with cuddles and kisses and strong approval. When he finds that his other devices do not get him any attention then he may stop it.

Why do children wet their beds?

About 10% of the boys do it. If he has started going to school and is still wetting his bed, then he is labelled as bed wetter. It is known to run in families. Wetting may disturb the child and cause problem. Such a child needs understanding and co-operation, not 'blame'. When a child finds that his parents are helping him then he can cope with the problem easily.

A bed made with a detachable draw sheet over a plastic protective sheet on the bottom helps. Do not try to alter the child's feeding habits and please avoid punishment.

Who are the timid children?

Some children are shy and refuse to leave their mothers' sight and need help continuously. Younger infants may behave like this. In such cases, the mother herself may be very timid and fearful. Or she may be unduly possessive, over protective.

Who is a turbulent child?

One who always seems to be in trouble. A child who gets involved in fights, shouts, cries more easily, argues more furiously can be called a turbulent child. Such a child exhausts his parent easily.

All children are turbulent sometimes. But if your child was a handful virtually from birth and faffles you by crying then you may need a doctor to help your turbulent child.

Who can be called a difficult child?

Though destructive, noisy, given to tears and tantrums, a difficult child is generally highly intelligent and very affectionate. Such a child is very responsive too. Such children need more than average share of attention and expressed love. They need it because they doubt their own value. A clever parent never forgets the child's need.

How does the father of a turbulent child behave?

The father generally accuses his wife of spoiling their son. He may also fear that other children in the family may be neglected in favour of more difficult one. So the mother has not only to live with a difficult child but must help her husband to live with the child as well. The child, in such cases, desperately needs his father's support and may grow up to become a considerable achiever.

Physiology of Sex

Dr. L. C. Gupta

What about the physiology of sexuality between 1 to 1½ years?

The first year has been identified by Freud as the oral stage of psycho-sexual development. The mouth is the main channel of gratification. The infant needs a warm physical relationship with the mother if sensory and affectionate awakening is to be developed. Otherwise there are chances that he will have retarded sexual development, aggressive behaviour and socio-emotional problem.

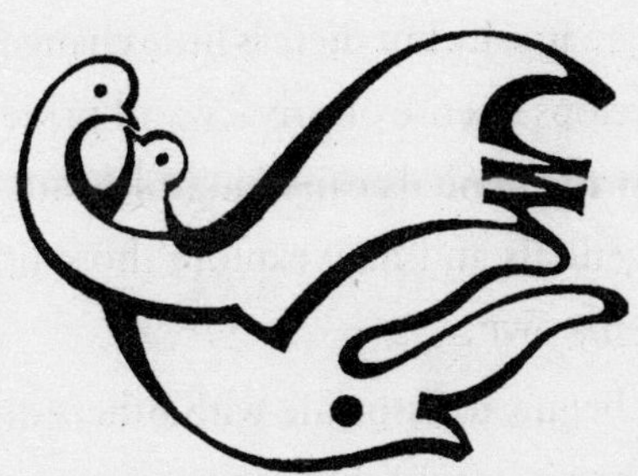

What psycho-social influences affect the sexuality?

Parentral treatment of males and females differ begining in the first few weeks of life. The daughters are handled gently while father treats boys roughly. Mothers appear to be more affectionate with their daughters. Such behaviour affects subsequent gender role behaviour. Pink rooms, dolls, delicate dresses, neatness and cleanliness have been traditionally associated with the feminine gender.

What happens at the age of 2 years?

The child learns neuromuscular coordination. Freud has designated

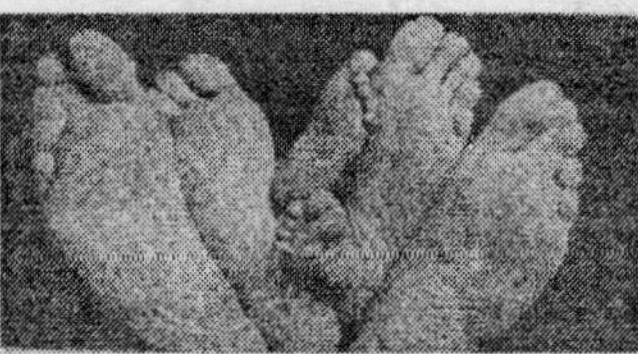

it as anal period. The child learns to associate his genitals with privacy. The parents discourage direct genital manipulation but a 2 year old obtains sensual, erotic sensation from being hugged and kissed by the family members as well as from rhythmic motor activities such as swinging and riding a toy horse.

What happens between the ages of 3-5 years?

The size of the body increases dramatically but there is little change in genital organs. The child develops a sense of privacy and pride in his genital. He discovers that the genitals can bring pleasure. The child enjoys fondling his genitals and may explore those of his playmates as well as exhibit his own.

At the end of 3 years, a child begins to associate with others of his own age and gradually becomes aware of differences between the two sexes. Attention is now directed to genitals of both sexes and there develops an urge to perform a sexual act. They start kissing and hugging. Boys and girls may be fascinated about each others' bathroom activities.

Children at this stage become curious to know where babies come from and how they get out of the stomach.

What should parents do at this stage?

Quality of communication between the parents and the child concerning sexual behaviour is very vital. If the parents are too strict and embarrass the child, the child may attach guilt to the pleasure associated with genitals.

What will happen if parents start threatening the child?

If parents threaten the child with 'We will cut off your hand if you don't stop playing with yourself' or worse 'Your penis will fall off if you play with it', the child will develop anxiety about loosing something dear. Such children may develop neurotic problems related to sex in adult age.

During this age, casual nudity of the parents of opposite sex may be deterimental to the young child.

What is mild sex play?

Mild sex play such as exhibiting one's genitals or inspecting of other children genitals is common while playing the role of a doctor. The child may lie on the top of other. Even when the children undress the activity includes nothing more than genital opposition.

How do children behave between the age of 8-9 years?

By this age interest in sexual exploration is less common than at the age of 6 years. But the interest and curiosity about reproduction

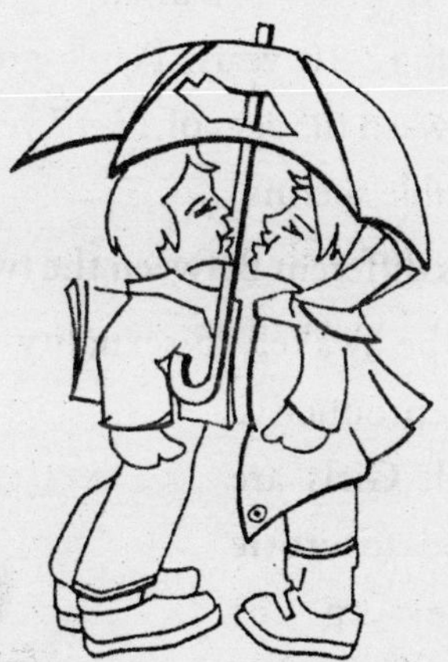

continues. Girls become interested in menstruation. Boys and girls start playing separately but their interest in the opposite sex continues in the form of preparing sex jokes etc. Both the sexes become conscious of their attractiveness. Kissing girls or teasing about boy friends and girl friends may take place during mixed play.

What happens during the age of 10-12 years?

Between 10-12 years there is an increased preoccupation with the changes taking place in one's body.

Do real changes take place between 13-15 years?

Yes, this is the period of acclerated growth and development of secondary sex characters. Girls may start menstruation. First few menstruations are not necessarily accompanied by ovulation. Girls may have ambivalent feelings towards their genitalia and menses may elicit negative feelings since it is a constant reminder of the reproductive consequences of sexual activity.

Estrogen causes increased growth of external genitalia.

In boys, the growth of pubic hair and enlargement of testicles begins at the age of 12-16 years. Penile growth and ability to ejaculate occurs between the ages of 13-17 years. First ejaculation may not contain viable sperms.

Are sexual activities different between the two genders?

A girl is slower to be awaken to sexuality than a boy. In girls sexual wishes and reproductive fears are confused. Girls are usually introduced to erotic feelings by petting or stimulation by a boy rather than by masturbation. Now a days more girls are becoming liberal and they fantasize without shame to organ.

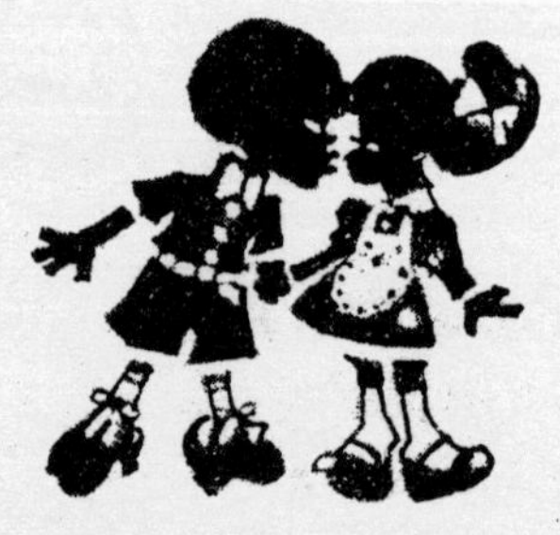

The first coital experience as regards physical pleasure is concerned is always disappointing unless orgasm occurs. The girl experiences more satisfaction in submission with a few feelings of guilt, shame, anxiety and disgust.

When girls and boys reach their sexual peak?

In girls there is no sudden increase in sexual activity at puberty as in case of boys. The girls show steady increase in sexual responsiveness and reach its peak at the age of 32.

Boys show a quick upsurge of sexual activity and reach at peak at the age of 18.

Sex dreams are a very small part of sexual outlet.

What is the sexual pattern between the age of 16-20 years?

Premarital intercourse has increased in both sexes. Girls may be concerned about unintended pregnancy. Becoming pregnant will affect their reputation and marriage aspects. During this period a mother should maintain a close relationship with her daughter to know her activities in order to avoid humiliation to the family.

> A woman begins by resisting a man's advances and ends up blocking his retreat.

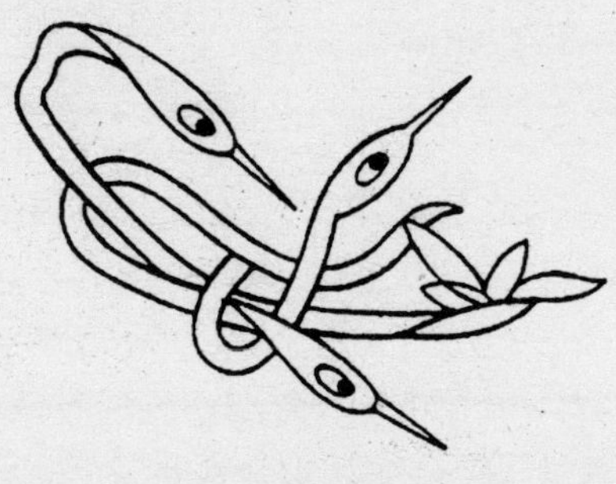

Nutrition During Pregnancy

Dr. Vandana Mangal
Mrs. Mani Mangal

The object of maternity care is to ensure that every expectant and nursing mother maintains good health and bears healthy children.

How does poor nourishment affect the outcome of pregnancy?

A poorly nourished woman is more likely to have complications during pregnancy and to bear a small infant in poor physical condition.

What factors may result in a low birth weight infant and increased mortality rate?

Factors include

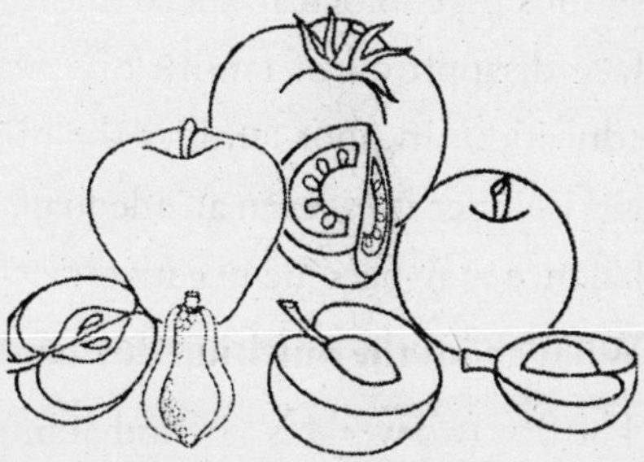

- High parity
- Small stature of mother
- Biological immaturity (under 17 years of age)
- Poverty
- Low pregnancy weight for height
- Smoking or taking certain drugs
- Unfavourable social environment

What is the relationship between nutrition and brain development?

The brain develops rapidly in a fetus and in the early postnatal period. Malnutrition during pregnancy and in the first weeks of life leads to reduced cell numbers and reduced brain weight. Once the increase in cell numbers is impaired, there is no reversal even if very rich diet is provided later on.

If malnutrition occurs during the third stage of growth, cells don't achieve their full size. But size of cells may improve once good diet is made available.

Does malnutrition affect behaviour also?

The development of brain and the resulting behaviour are dependent upon interaction of genetic and environmental factors including nutrition, illness, psychological factors and cultural patterns. An undernourished child is always irritable.

What are the risks to an adolescent pregnant girl?

In addition to physical risks, the pregnant adolescent often has serious psychological, social and economic problems. She has to face disapproval of family. She may be unable to continue her education. In poor families she may be poorly nourished. If the girl is under stress even an adequate diet, the calcium and nitrogen balance may become negative.

What about the nutrition during the first 2 weeks of pregnancy?

The first two weeks is a period of implantation. During this period, the fertilized ovum becomes embedded in the uterine wall. At this time the fetus is nourished from the outer layer of germ plasm and from secretions of uterine gland.

What type of nutrition is required between 2 and 6 weeks?

This period is known as the period of organogenesis. During this time nourishment is obtained from blood. But riboflavin deficiency is associated with poor skeletal formation. Pyridoxine deficiency results in neuromotor problems. While vitamin B_{12} deficiency results in hydrocephalus; niacin and folic deficiency may cause a cleft palate.

What happens in the last 7 months?

The last 7 months are known as the growth period. During this stage the placenta develops and takes over its role of giving nutrition to the fetus. Its weight varies from 350 to 1000 gram. Placenta allows passage of folacin, iron and vitamin C.

What is the requirement of calories?

The total calorie requirement of producing the fetus, the placenta, other maternal tissue and establishing reserve is about 80,000 kcal.

For most women an extra allowance of 300 kcal daily will serve the purpose.

What will be the maximum requirement of calories during pregnancy?

Calorie requirement may vary as much as 600 to 750 calories extra depending upon the activity of the woman. A woman responsible for full household duties may require more than 300, calories extra per day.

Is a calorie restriction needed for an obese woman?

Restriction of calories is no longer advocated although obesity may increase the risk of pregnancy. But a woman taking lower calories will have lower glucose level resulting in lower glycogenesis and increased ketosis. Ketosis may impair neurological development.

How much of extra protein is required in pregnancy?

About 925 gram proteins are deposited in the fetus and the maternal tissues during pregnancy. Protein may be stored in the body at a uniform rate during the entire pregnancy.

Recommended allowance during pregnancy is an extra 30 grams daily.

Does requirement of calcium also increase during pregnancy?

The full term fetus contains about 28 gram calcium. Some calcium and phosphorus deposition takes place in early pregnancy, but most of calcification of bones occurs during the last 2 months of pregnancy. The first set of teeth begins to form about the 8th week of the prenatal life and they are all formed by the end of the prenatal period. Hence a woman should increase her consumption of calcium.

How much extra iron is needed?

The amount of iron in a full term fetus is about 300 mg. For increased blood and maternal tissues, an additional 500 mg is required.

To cover this 3.5 mg iron must be absorbed daily.

How much iodine is needed?

The daily allowance of 175 μg iodine is easily met by using iodized salt.

Does the need for sodium also increase?

During pregnancy requirement of sodius also increases due to the enlarging maternal tissues and expanding blood volume.

Is any specific diet required during morning sickness?

Early morning nausea may be overcome by the use of high carbohydrate foods like jelly, sweets and cake before getting up from bed. Fluids should be taken between meals.

What diet will be useful during constipation?

Constipation generally develops in the later half of pregnancy. Limited exercise and insufficient bulk in diet may cause constipation. Whole grain cereals, fruits and vegetables rich in fiber will be useful. Adequate fluid should be taken.

What is pica?

Pica is a practice of eating non food items, clay, starch etc. among pregnant women. There is no scientific basis for this craving.

What about alcohol consumption during pregnancy?

Women consuming two or three drinks per day have children weighing considerably less and have less power of sucking. These children often fail to catch up in growth even by 5 years of age.

Can a pregnant lady consume caffeine?

Caffeine crosses through the placenta to the fetus rapidly, so a pregnant woman is advised not to consume caffeine in large quantities.

LACTATION

Every woman produces 750-850 ml of milk. So it is obvious that the requirement for protein, minerals, calories becomes more during lactation than during pregnancy.

What will be the requirement of calories?

80-95 calories are required to produce 100 ml of milk. For an average daily production of 800 ml about 650 calories will be required.

Fat deposits during pregnancy will furnish 200-300 kcal for the first 100 days of lactation. Thus an added 500 kcal in the daily diet is advised.

How much of extra proteins will be required?

Each 100 ml. of human milk contains 1.2 gram of proteins. So about 10 gram of protein will be required. The need for protein is greatest when lactation has reached its maximum.

What will be the requirement of minerals?

Calcium reserves have to be developed during pregnancy itself and 4-5 cups of milk daily is recommended during lactation.

An infant is born with a large reserve of iron since milk is not a good source of iron. Iron rich foods are essential for mother and child too.

Are some extra vitamins needed during lactation?

Mother's diet should be sufficient in vitamin B_6. Ascorbic acid is transferred to the milk and the needs of the infant are fully met if the mother's diet is adequate.

What are the calorie requirement of infants?

A baby needs 120 calories per kg of body weight. During 1-2 years the baby's need increases to 1000 calories. It comes to nearly 50% of food what his mother eats. After the age of 1 year, practically 100 calories more will be required.

How many proteins will be required?

Proteins are required for growth and maintenance of the body. Each gram of protein provides 4.1 calories equivalent of carbohydrates. Animal proteins are complete proteins while vegetable proteins are incomplete ones lacking in one or two aminoacids. But if you combine different vegetable proteins it comes to near about complete proteins.

Calories and protein requirement

Age group	**Calories** per kg body weight	**Proteins** grams per kg
0-6 months	108	2.0
6-12 months	98	1.65
Daily requirement from 6 months to 1 year		
1-3 years	1240	22
4-6 years	1700	30

What are the calories requirement of children of different ages?

Age	Boys	Girls
1+	1095	1080
2+	1300	1200
3+	1460	1310
4+	1530	1460
5+	1775	1640
6+	1775	1640
7+	2030	1860
8+	2040	1890
9+	2160	1850
10+	2180	1910

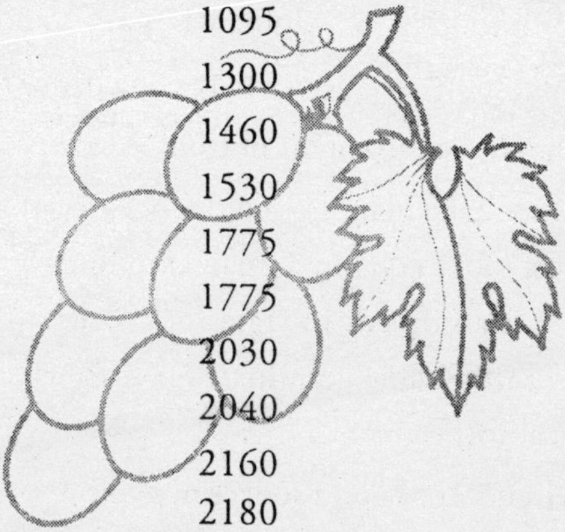

Values are in approximation.

What is a balanced diet?

A balanced diet is a diet which provides sufficient calories, proteins fats, carbohydrates, minerals and to keep something in reserve to meet the body's requirement during lean periods.

Balanced diet for infants and young children

	6-12 months gm/day	1-3 years gm/day
Cereals	45	120
Pulses	15	30
Milk	500 ml	500 ml
Root vegetables	50	50
Green leafy vegetables	25	50
Other vegetables	25	50
Fruits	100	100
Sugar	25	25
Fats/oil	10	20

Fats give 9 calories per gram more than the double provided by carbohydrates and proteins. Fats improve palatability of food and facilitate absorption of fat soluble vitamins A and D.

About 20 to 30% of calories may come from fats.

What will be the requirement of iron?

Iron is used to make hemoglobin. Deficiency of this may lead to anemia. Most foods contain a small amount of iron and hardly 5 to 15% of it is absorbed. Phytates of cereals, tea, coffee hinder absorption of iron while germinated cereals, vitamin C, oranges increases its absorption.

What food items are a good source of iron?

Green leafy vegetables, gur or jaggery (sugarcane) are good sources of iron.

Dietary iron requirement in mg/day

	Iron mg			Iron mg
Men	28	Child	1-3 years	12
Women	30		4-6 years	18
Pregnant women	38		7-9 years	26
Lactating women	30	Adolescents		28

What is the need of zinc?

A child needs zinc to grow normally. Zinc deficiency may cause slow growth, slow healing of wounds, poor appetite and persistent diarrhoea. Body requires 4 to 6 mg zinc daily. Cereals, pulses, meat, all contain zinc so deficiency in the real sense hardly develops. But recovery is faster if zinc is given along with ORS in case of diarrhoea.

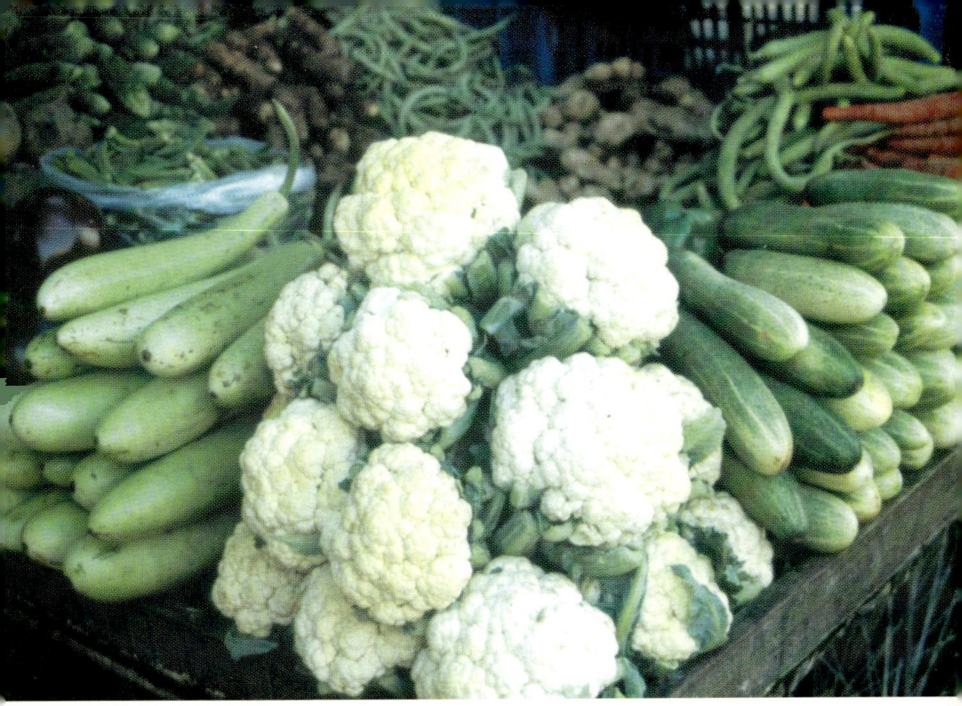

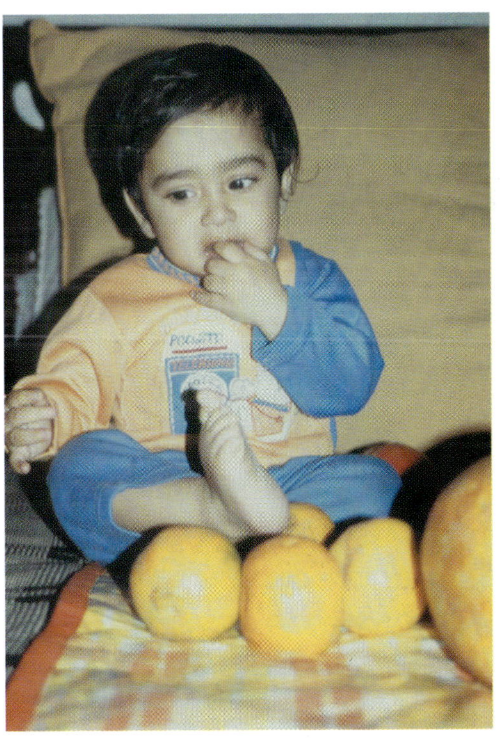

Provide mixed eatables to children.

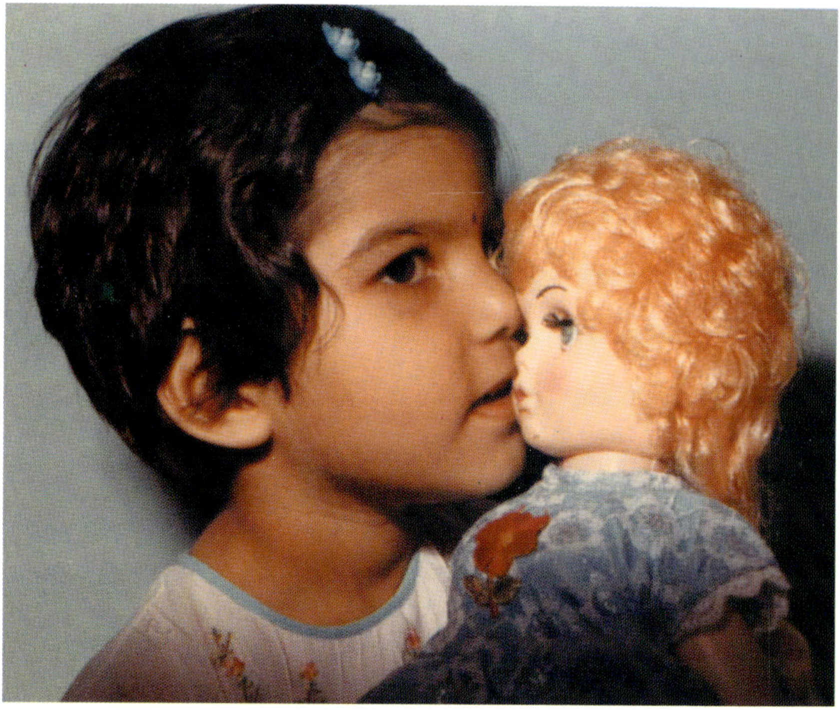

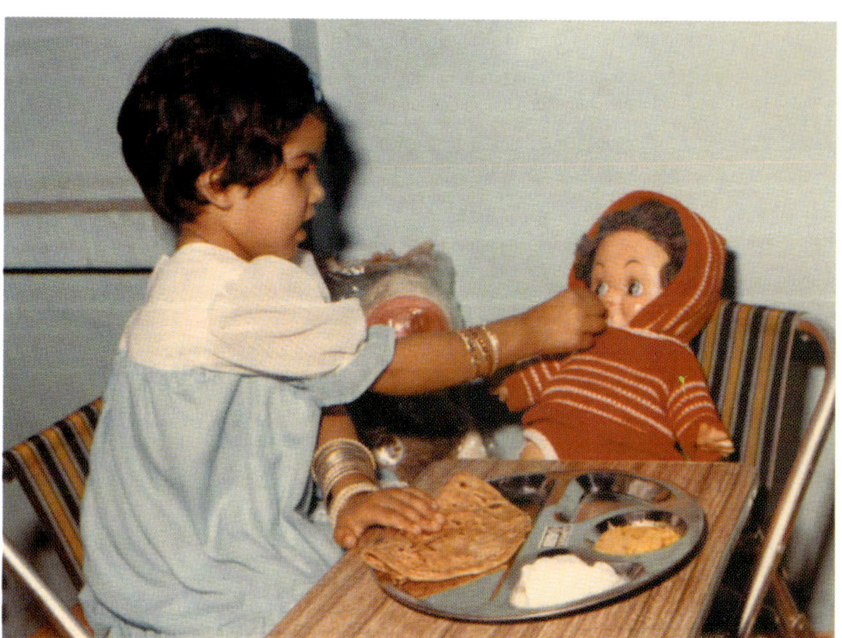

Dolls are the best friends of girls.

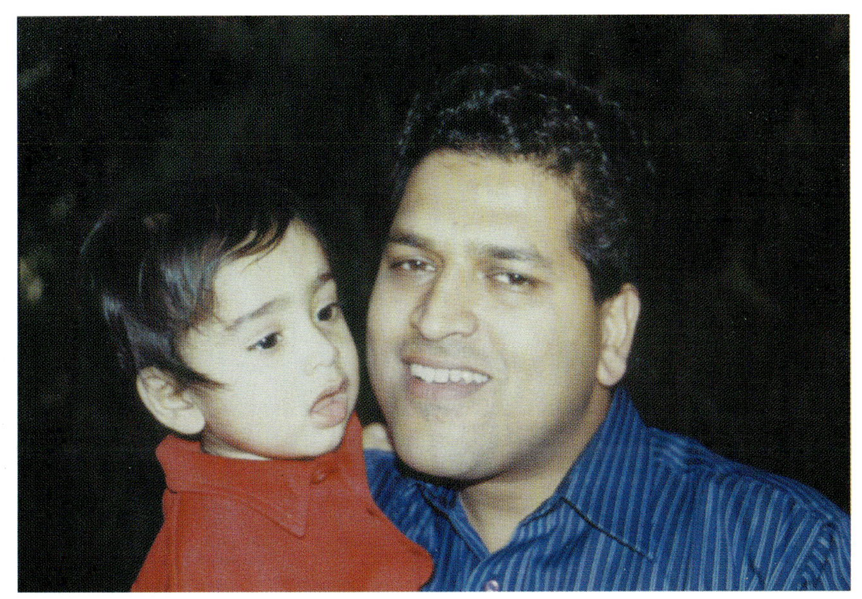

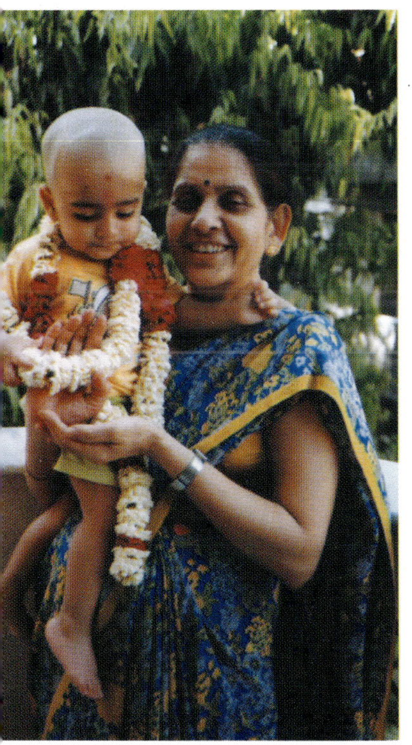

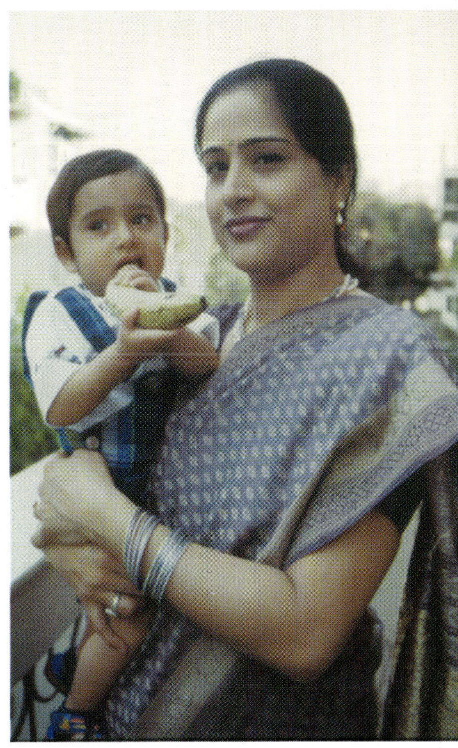

Children enjoy the company of their parents.

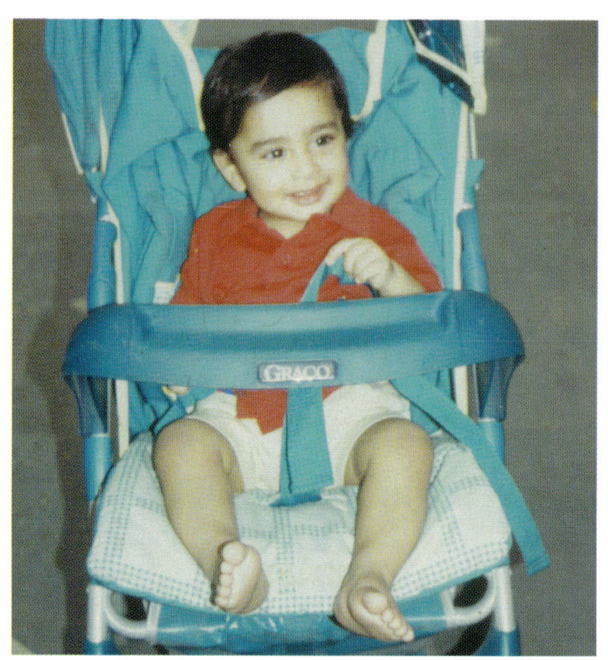

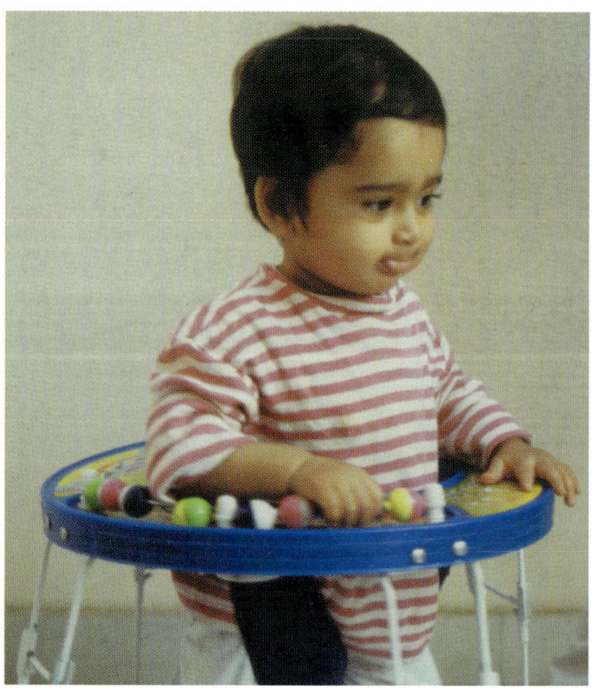

Children loves to be mobile.

Balanced Diet

A balanced diet takes care of the nutrients required by the body + provides for a little reserve to meet the requirement in case of lean periods.

Balanced diet for different sex and age group (Grams)

Food Item	Adult Man			Adult Woman			Boys	Girls	Children	
	Sedentary Work	Moderate Work	Heavy Work	Sedentary Work	Moderate Work	Heavy Work	10-12 yrs	10-12 yrs	1-3 yrs	4-6 yrs
Cereals	460	520	670	410	440	575	420	380	175	270
Pulses	40	50	60	40	45	50	45	45	35	35
Leafy vegetables	40	40	40	100	100	50	50	50	40	50
Other vegetables	60	70	80	40	40	100	50	50	20	30
Roots and tubers	50	60	80	50	50	60	30	30	10	20
Milk	150	200	250	100	150	200	250	250	300	250
Oil and fat	40	45	65	20	25	40	40	35	15	25
Sugar or jaggery	30	35	55	20	20	40	45	45	30	40

Suggested substitution for non-vegetarians

Food items which can be deleted from non-vegetarian diet	Substitution than can be suggested for deleted item or items
5% of pulses (20– 30 gm)	1. One egg or 30 gm of meat or fish. 2. Addition 5 gm of fat or oil.
10% of pulses (40–60 gm)	1. Two eggs or 50 gm of meat or fish or one egg + 30 gm of meat or fish 2. 10 gm of fat or oil.

Additional allowances during pregnancy and lactation

Food Items	During Pregnancy	Calories (Kcal)	During Lactation	Calories (Kcal)
Cereal	35 gm	118	60 gm	203
Pulses	15 gm	52	30 gm	105
Milk	100 gm	83	100 gm	83
Fat	–	–	10 gm	90
Sugar	10 gm	40	10 gm	40
Total		293		521

FOOD FOR PRE-SCHOOL CHILDREN

What about food habits and development?

Food continues to be a major part throughout the growing period. Actually food is a means of communication. It has social and cultural meaning too.

Food habits are a part of a satisfying human relationship and contribute to social and personal enjoyment.

What should be the diet?

Toddlers have a short attention span and are easily distracted from eating. Their response to food is always inconsistent. Their eating behaviour is messy.

During the second year child eats low, corresponding to the slower rate of growth. The child reduces his milk intake at about 9 months but start to increase again between the 1 and 2 years. Some children's appetite improve by 5 years of age. Mothers should understand that the child will remain well nourished provided foods of high nutrient density are offered.

Do children like highly flavoured food?

Children have high taste sensitivity, they prefer mildly flavoured food. Plain food is preferred to mixtures. They don't like extremes of food temperature.

Does the feel of the food affect child?

The feel of the food is important to young children. They enjoy food which can be picked up by their fingers like potato chips, banana etc. The ability to chew food should determine the texture of food. Children are fond of different fruits.

Do children develop food faddism?

Food fads are not uncommon between 2 and 4 years of age. A

child may dislike all but a few foods. But such occurences do not last long.

How to develop good food habits?

Meals should be served at a regular interval in a pleasant environment. A deep plate and a blunt spoon of good quality melamine should be used. Cup should be partially filled to avoid spilling.

Children like colourful foods. Their appetite differ from day to day. Even favourite foods should not be given too often. Encouragement and praise are helpful but favourite foods should not be used as a bribe or reward.

DIET FOR THE SCHOOL GOING CHILD

School children are generally better fed. Group acceptance is important. Child wants to keep up with classmates. At school he gets acquainted with food patterns different from his home. He learns that certain foods are acceptable to the peer group.

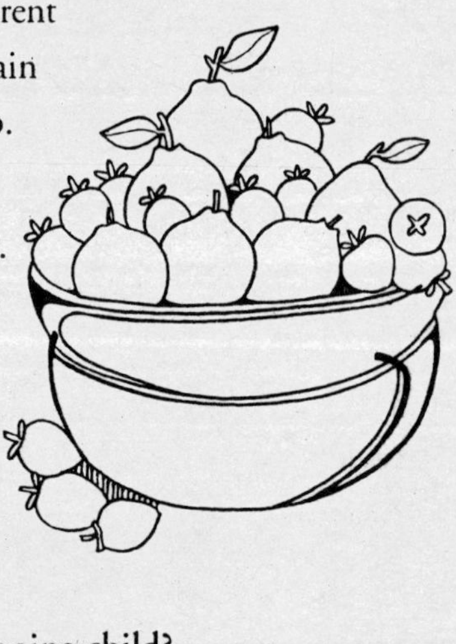

Do school children have dislikes?

School children have a few dislikes, e.g. for some vegetables which are not eaten in good amount.

During 8-10 years of age the appetite increases. Most children remain in a hurry and do not want to give time for meals. They try to miss breakfast.

What about the appetite of a school going child?

School children are subject to many stresses which affect their appetite. Communicable diseases reduce the appetite on the one hand while increasing the body's needs on the other. School work, class competition and emotional stress have adverse effect on appetite.

Why do certain children become obese?

It is a form of overnutrition. Childhood or juvenile onset of obesity is refractory to treatment and tends to persist into adulthood. Overconcerned parents unwittingly establish pattern of overeating when they introduce solid foods.

The syndrome of a pale, flabby child sitting in an airconditioned room infront of a television eating something or the other is indicative of the child becoming obese.

What is the role of 'Junk food'?

Junk food includes items of fast food restaurant, chips, cakes, sweets, soft drinks. These may lack in essential nutrients. These are oily preparations supplying high calories. Most fast food meals are low in fiber, vitamins A & C, folacin and some trace minerals.

Can a child be maintained on a vegetarian diet?

Why not? Children can be nourished satisfactorily on a lacto-ovo vegetarian diet. Only thing that should be kept in mind is the fact that the diet should be one of mixed cereals, pulses and vegetables.

What is emphasis required if vegetarian diet is to be given?

Following points require emphasis

- Sufficient calories to meet growth as well as activity requirement.

- Inclusion of food which complement each other for aminoacid. For example wheat flour may be mixed with gramflour. Wheat lacks in lysine while besan lacks in methionine. Mixture complements each other.
- Supplementation with calcium, zinc and vitamin B_{12} is required.

Food Values

Food values per 100 gm edible portion (ICMR : 1971)

Food	Protein gm	Fat gm	Calcium mg	Iron mg	Vit'C' mg	Vit'A' mg	Calories
RICE							
Raw milled	6.8	0.5	10	3.1	0	0	345
Parboiled	6.4	0.4	9	4.0	0	0	346
Flakes	6.6	1.2	20	20.0	0	0	346
Puffed	7.5	0.1	20	6.6	0	0	325
WHEAT							
Whole flour	12.1	1.7	48	11.5	0	29	341
Flour refined	11.0	0.9	23	2.5	0	25	348
Suji	10.4	0.8	16	1.6	0	-	348
Bread white	7.8	0.7	11	1.1	0	0	245
MILLETS							
Bajra	11.6	5.0	42	5.0	0	132	361
Jowar	10.4	1.9	25	5.8	0	47	349
Maize	11.1	3.6	10	2.0	0	90	342
Ragi	7.3	1.3	344	6.4	0	42	328
PULSES DALS							
Bengal gram	20.8	5.6	56	9.1	1	129	372
Black gram	24.0	1.4	154	9.1	0	38	347
Green gram	24.5	1.2	75	8.5	0	49	348
Red gram	22.3	1.7	73	5.8	0	132	335
WHOLE DAL							
Bengal gram	17.1	5.3	202	10.2	3	189	360
Green gram	24.0	1.3	127	7.3	0	92	334
Lentil (masur)	25.0	0.7	69	4.8	0	294	343
Peas dry	19.7	1.1	75	5.1	0	39	315
Rajmah	22.9	1.3	260	5.8	0	-	346
Moth beans	23.6	1.1	202	9.5	0	9	330
Soya bean	43.2	19.5	240	11.5	0	426	432

Food	Protein gm	Fat gm	Calcium mg	Iron mg	Vit'C' mg	Vit'A' mg	Calories
NUTS & SEEDS							
Groundnut	25.3	40.1	90	2.8	0	37	567
Sesame	18.3	43.0	1450	10.5	0	60	563
Poppy seeds	21.7	19	1584	-	-	-	408
Cashewnut	21.2	47	50	5.0	-	-	596
Almond	20.8	59	230	4.5	-	-	655
Dry coconut	6.8	62	40	2.7	7	-	662
MILK AND MILK PRODUCTS							
Milk cow	3.2	4.1	120	0.2	2	174	67
Milk buffalo	4.3	8.8	210	0.2	1	160	117
Milk goat	3.3	4.5	170	0.3	1	182	72
Curd	3.1	4.0	149	0.2	1	102	60
Butter milk	0.8	1.1	30	0.8	-	0	30
Cheese	24.1	25.1	790	2.1	-	-	348
Khoa	14.6	31.2	650	5.8	-	-	421
Whole milk Powder	25.8	26.7	950	0.6	4	1400	496
Skimmed Milk powder	38.0	0.1	1370	1.4	5	0	357
EGG & MEAT							
Egg hen	13.3	13.3	60	2.1	0	600	173
Mutton	18.5	13.3	150	2.5	-	0	194
Goat meat	21.4	3.6	12	-	-	-	118
Chicken	26.0	0.6	25	-	-	-	109
Beef	22.6	2.6	10	0.8	2	0	114
Pork	18.7	4.4	30	2.2	2	0	114
Liver sheep	19.3	7.5	10	6.3	20	0	150
FISH							
Pomfrets	17.0	1.3	200	0.9	-	-	87
Hilsa	21.8	19.4	180	2.1	24	-	273
Prawn fresh	19.1	1.0	323	5.3	-	-	89
Fish fresh	11.2	5.8	240	2.3	-	-	138
Fish dry	5.5	2.7	315	3.5	-	-	255
Crab	8.9	1.1	1370	21.2	-	-	59

Food	Protein gm	Fat gm	Calcium mg	Iron mg	Vit'C' mg	Vit'A' mg	Calories
GREEN LEAFY VEGETABLES							
Amranth	4.0	0.5	397	25.5	99	5520	45
Bathua	3.7	0.4	150	4.2	35	1700	30
Cabbage	1.8	0.1	39	0.8	124	1200	27
Colocasia Green leaves	3.9	1.5	227	10.0	12	10270	56
Coriander	3.3	0.6	184	18.5	135	6918	44
Drumstick Leaves	6.7	1.7	440	7.0	220	6780	92
Fenegreek	4.4	0.9	395	16.5	52	2300	49
Lettuce	2.1	0.3	50	2.4	10	990	21
Radish Leaves	3.8	0.4	265	3.6	81	5300	28
Spinach	2.0	0.7	73	10.9	28	5580	26
BULBS & TUBERS							
Beetroot	1.7	0.1	18	1.0	10	0	43
Carrot	0.9	0.2	80	2.2	3	1890	48
Radish	0.7	0.1	35	0.4	15	0	17
Onion	1.2	0.1	47	0.7	2	0	50
Potato	1.6	0.1	10	0.7	17	0	97
Colocasia	3.0	0.1	40	1.7	0	-	97
Yam	1.2	0.1	50	0.6	0	260	79
OTHER VEGETABLES							
Drumstick	2.5	0.1	30	5.3	120	110	26
Capsicum	1.2	0.3	10	1.0	137	420	24
Bitter gourd	1.6	0.2	20	1.8	88	125	25
Beans French	1.7	0.1	50	1.7	24	130	26
Beans cluster	3.2	0.4	130	4.5	49	200	60
Peas	7.2	0.3	20	1.5	9	80	93

Food	Protein gm	Fat gm	Calcium mg	Iron mg	Vit'C' mg	Vit'A' mg	Calories
FRUITS							
Amla	0.5	0.1	50	1.2	600	9	58
Guava	0.9	0.3	10	1.4	212	0	51
Grape	0.7	0.1	20	0.2	31	0	32
Lemon	1.0	0.9	70	2.3	39	0	57
Mosambi	0.8	0.3	40	0.7	50	0	43
Orange	0.7	0.2	26	0.3	30	1104	65
Lichi	1.1	0.2	10	0.7	31	0	61
Melon	0.3	0.2	32	1.4	26	170	17
Papaya	0.6	0.1	17	0.5	57	665	32
Pineapple	0.4	0.1	20	1.2	39	++	46
Sitaphal	1.6	0.4	17	1.5	37	0	104
Strawberry	0.7	0.2	30	1.8	52	15	44
Tomato	0.9	0.2	48	0.4	27	350	20
Apple	0.2	0.5	10	1.0	1	0	59
Bael Fruit	1.8	0.3	85	0.6	3	55	137
Banana	1.2	0.3	17	0.9	7	78	116
Cherries	1.1	0.5	24	1.3	7		64
Figs	1.3	0.2	80	1.0	5	162	37
Jack fruit	1.9	0.1	20	0.5	7	175	88
Mango	0.6	0.4	14	1.3	16	2740	74
Chiku	0.7	0.1	28	2.0	6	95	98

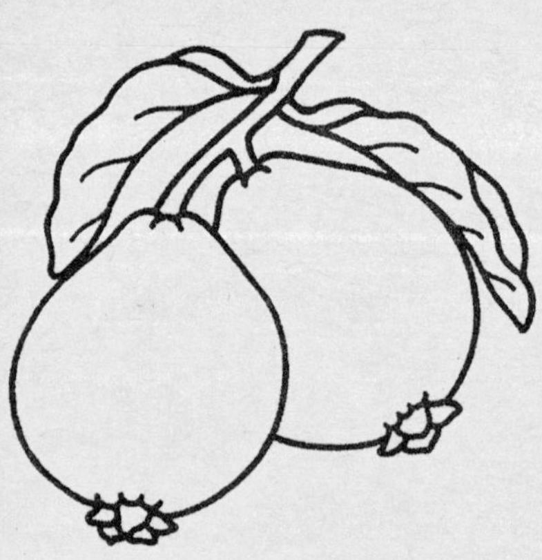

Vitamin Contents of Foods

Food	Carotene (µg)	Thiamine (mg)	Riboflavin (mg)	Niacin (mg)	Folic Acid (mg)	Vitamin 'C' (mg)
GRAINS						
Bajra	132	0.33	0.25	2.3	45.5	0
Jowar	47	0.37	0.13	3.1	20.0	0
Maize, dry	90	0.42	0.10	1.8	20.0	0
Maize, tender	32	0.11	0.17	0.6	-	6
Rice, parboiled	-	0.27	0.12	4.0	-	0
Rice, raw (milled)	0	0.06	0.06	3.9	-	77
Samai	0	0.30	0.09	3.2	9.0	
Wheat flour	29	0.49	0.17	5.5	36.6	-
PULSES						
Bengal gram	189	0.30	0.15	2.9	186.0	3
Bengal gram dal	129	0.48	0.18	2.4	147.5	1
Black gram	38	0.42	0.20	2.0	132.0	0
Green gram	94	0.47	0.27	2.1	-	0
Horee gram	71	0.42	0.20	1.5	-	1
Math beans	9	0.45	0.09	1.5	-	2
Peas	83	0.25	0.01	0.8	-	9
Red gram dal	469	0.32	0.33	3.0	-	25
Soya bean	426	0.73	0.39	3.2	103	0
LEAFY VEGETABLES						
Amaranth	5400	0.21	0.09	1.2	-	169
Cabbage	120	0.06	0.09	0.4	-	72
Carrot leaves	5700	0.04	0.37	2.1	-	79
Colocasia leaves	12000	0.06	0.45	1.9	-	63
Fenugreek	2340	0.04	0.31	0.8	-	220
Lettuce	990	0.09	0.13	0.50	-	10
Curry leaves	7560	0.08	.21	2.3	93.9	4
Mustard leaves	2622	0.03	-	-	-	33
Radish leave	5295	0.18	0.47	0.8	-	81
Spinach	5580	0.03	0.03	0.26	123	28
Turnip green	9396	0.31	0.57	5.4	180	-

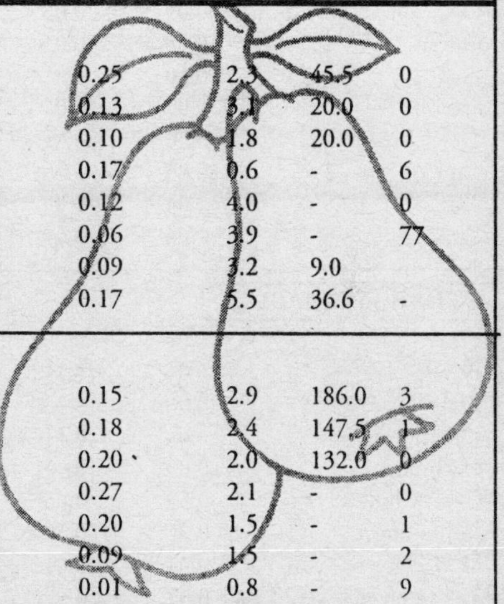

Food	Carotene (µg)	Thiamine (mg)	Riboflavin (mg)	Niacin (mg)	Folic Acid	Vitamin 'C' (mg)
ROOTS AND TUBERS						
Beetroot	0	0.04	0.09	0.4	-	1
Carrot	1890	0.04	0.02	0.6	15.0	3
Colocasia	24	0.09	0.03	0.4	-	10
Onion	0	0.08	0.01	0.4	6	11
Potato	24	0.10	0.01	1.2	0	16
Radish	4	0.02	0.03	1.4	-	21
Sweet Potato	3	0.06	0.03	0.7	-	24
Tapico	-	0.05	0.10	0.3	-	25
Turnip	0	0.04	0.04	0.5	-	43
Yarn	260	0.06	0.07	0.7	-	0
OTHER VEGETABLES						
Bitter gourd	123	0.07	0.09	0.5	-	88
Brinjal	74	0.04	0.11	0.9	34.0	12
Broad beans	9	0.08	-	0.8		12
Cauliflower	30	0.04	0.11	0.9	34	52
Cucumber	0	0.03	0	0.2	14.7	7
Gaint Chillies	427	0.55	0.05	0.1	137	-
Ladies finger	52	0.07	0.10	0.6	105	13
Mango green	90	0.04	0.01	0.2	-	3
Papaya green	0	0.01	0.01	0.1	-	12
Pumpkin	50	0.06	0.04	0.5	13.1	2
Tomato	192	0.07	0.01	0.4	-	31
Tinda	13	0.08	0.08	0.5	-	12
NUTS & OIL SEEDS						
Almond	0	0.24	0.57	4.4	-	0
Cashew Nut	60	0.63	0.19	1.2	-	0
Coconut dry	0	0.08	0.01	3.0	16.5	7
Groundnut	37	0.90	0.13	19.9	20.0	224
Pista	144	0.67	0.28	2.3	-	-
Walnut	6	0.45	0.40	1.0	-	0
Gingelly seed	60	1.01	0.34	4.4	134	0
Linseed	30	0.23	0.07	1.0	-	0

Food	Carotene (µg)	Thiamine (mg)	Riboflavin (mg)	Niacin (mg)	Folic Acid	Vitamin 'C' (mg)
SPICES						
Chillies, dry	345	0.93	0.43	9.5	-	50
FRUITS						
Amla	9	0.03	0.01	0.2	-	600
Apricot	2160	0.04	0.13	0.6	-	6
Bael fruit	55	0.13	0.03	1.1	-	8
Dates, dried	26	0.01	0.02	0.9	-	3
Figs	162	0.06	0.05	0.6	-	5
Grapes	-	0.12	0.02	0.3	-	-
Guava	0	0.03	0.03	0.4	-	212
Jackfruit	175	0.03	0.03	0.3	-	7
Lemon	0	0.02	0.01	0.1	-	63
Mango ripe	2743	0.08	0.09	0.9		16
Orange juice	15	0.06	0.02	0.4	-	64
Papaya	666	0.04	0.25	0.2		4
Pears	28	0.06	0.03	0.2	-	0
Plum	166	0.04	0.1	0.3	-	5
Strawberry	18	0.03	0.02	0.2	-	52
Tomato	351	0.12	0.06	-	-	
Pineapple	18	0.20	0.12	0.1	-	39
FISH AND SEA FOODS						
Bhanger	-	-	-	1.8	-	-
Crab muscle	780	-	-	3.1	-	-
Koi	-	-	-	0.5	-	-
Lata	-	-	-	0.8	-	-
Mrigal	-	-	-	0.7	16.7	-
Prawn	0	0.01	0.10	4.8	-	-
Rohu	0.05	0.07	0.7	22		
Shrimp	-	-	-	-	18.6	-

Food	Carotene (µg)	Thiamine (mg)	Riboflavin (mg)	Niacin (mg)	Folic Acid	Vitamin 'C' (mg)
OTHER ANIMAL PRODUCTS						
Beef	345	0.93	0.43	9.5	-	50
Buffalo meat	-	-	-	7.8	-	-
Egg, hen	600	0.10	0.40	0.1	80	-
Goat meat	-	-	-	4.5	-	-
Liver, goat	-	-	-	176.2	-	-
Liver, sheep	-	0.36	1.70	17.6	188.0	20
Mutton	-	0.18	0.14	6.8	5.8	-
Pork	-	0.54	0.09	2.8	-	2
MILK AND MILK PRODUCTS						
Milk, buffalo	160	0.04	0.10	0.1	5.6	1
Milk, cow	174	0.05	0.19	0.1	8.5	2
Milk, human	137	0.02	0.02	1.3	3	-
Chenna	366	0.07	0.02	-	-	3
Cheese	273	-	-	-	-	-
Butter	3200	-	-	-	-	-
Ghee,cow milk	200	-	-	-	-	-
Ghee, buffalo milk	900	-	-	-	-	-

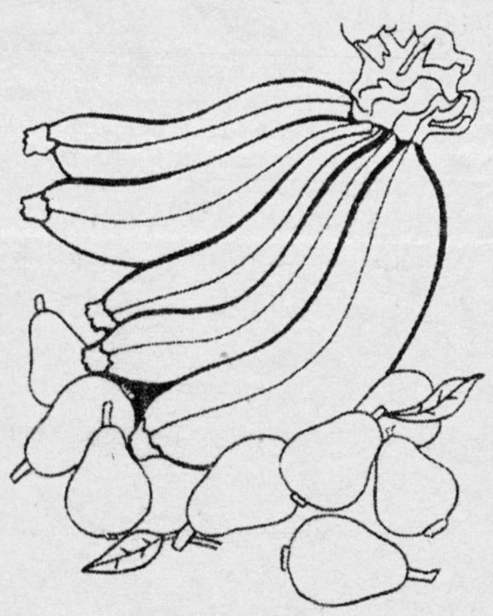

Mineral Contents of Foods (mg/100 gm)

Food	Magnesium	Sodium	Potassium	Manganese	Zinc
Maize	139	10.9	307	0.48	2.8
Rice, parboiled	61	-	-	0.66	1.33
Wheat,whole	138	17.1	284	2.29	2.7
Bengal gram	119	7.3	808	1.21	6.1
Black gram dal	130	39.8	800	0.96	3.0
Peas, green	34	7.8	79		
Rajmah	184			4.5	
Soyabean	238			2.35	4.4
Cabbage	31			0.18	0.30
Radish leaves	22			0.01	0.08
Spinach	64	58.4	181	0.56	0.30
Onion	16	4.0	127	0.18	0.41
Potato	30	11.0	247	0.13	0.53
Radish white	-	33.0	138	-	-
Bitter gourd	36	17.8	152	0.88	0.46
Cauliflower	18	53.0	138	0.10	0.10
Brinjal	15	3.0	200	0.13	0.22
Cucumber	14	10,2	50	0.14	0.23
Ladies finger	53	6.9	10.3	-	0.42
Mango, green	16	43.0	83	0.07	0.07
Pumpkin	38	5.6	139	0.05	0.26
Tinda	14	35.0	24	0.12	-
Tomato	15	45.8	114	0.19	-
Almonds	373	-	-	1.88	3.57
Cashewnut	349	-	-	1.42	5.99
Groundnut	-	-	-	.10	12.20
Walnut	302	-	-	2.32	
Garlic, dry	71	-	-	0.86	1.83
Amla fruit	-	5.6	225	-	-
Apple	7	28.0	75	0.14	0.06
Banana, ripe	41	36.6	88	-	-
Grapes	82	-	-	0.12	0.33
Lemon	19	-	270	0.07	-
Guava	24	5.5	91	0.11	-
Maize	24	-	-	0.14	0.16
Sweet lime			170		
Mango, ripe	270	26.0	205	0.13	0.27
Melon water	13	27.3	160	-	-

Food	Magnesium	Sodium	Potassium	Manganese	Zinc
Orange	9	4.5	9.3	-	-
Papaya	11	6.0	69	-	-
Pineapple	33	34.7	37	-	-
Tomato	-	12.9	146	0.26	0.41
Chingri, dried	-	Copper	1.40	-	-
Helsa	-	52.0	183	-	-
Rohu	13	101.0	288	-	-
Beef muscle	-	52.0	214	-	-
Liver, goat		73.0	160		
Mutton		33.0	270		
Milk, buffalo		19.0	90		
Milk, cow		73.0	140		
Curd		32.0	130		

In world there are two powers the sword and the spirit. The spirit has always vanquished the sword.

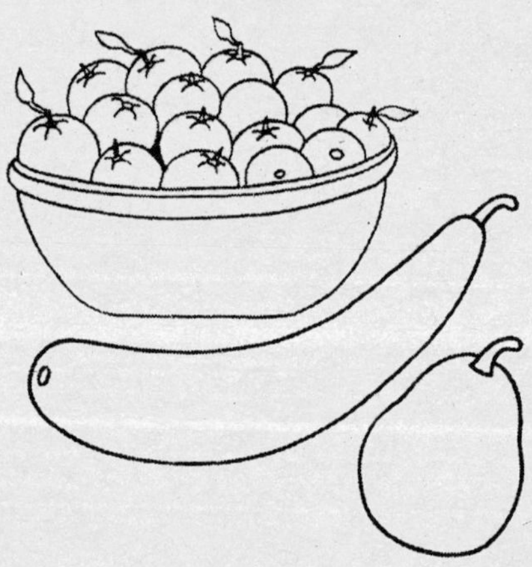

Miscellaneous Facts

Kusum Gupta
Mani Raj Sharma

STAMMERING

What is stammering?

Stammering is an involuntary repetition, prolongation or block which affects the normal flow of words. The child knows what to say, still even with his best efforts, words may not come out smoothly. It results in loss of self-confidence and frustration.

What should parents do when a child stammers?

Stammering could be due to physical, emotional or social influence.

- Create a calm and relaxed atmosphere when talking to a child.
- Instead of asking him to talk slowly, slow down your own speech. Then he will follow you.
- Use simple and short sentences while talking to your child.
- Maintain eye contact while talking to your child.
- Do not look away when he stammers.
- If needed consult a speech therapist.

PARENTS

What is the role of parents in producing aggressive child?

Lessons of good behaviour get confused when something breaks down in early socialization, when the brain is row. Parents who are overly punitive or set the wrong example with their own impulsive behaviour, have more aggressive children.

Should parents overlook a child's tantrum?

No, excusing aggression in early childhood means a child's path is set irrevocably toward deliquency, dropping out of school and crime. Intervention, it seems, needs to come sooner than ever. If aggressive children do not learn to control their anger early, they might never learn at all.

How parents affect a child's emotional development?

Children who live in orphanges or who spend their days in day nurseries wither in body, in intellect and in emotions. They never fully recover. Even a child of 6 months will lose his smile and appetite when his caretaker disappears.

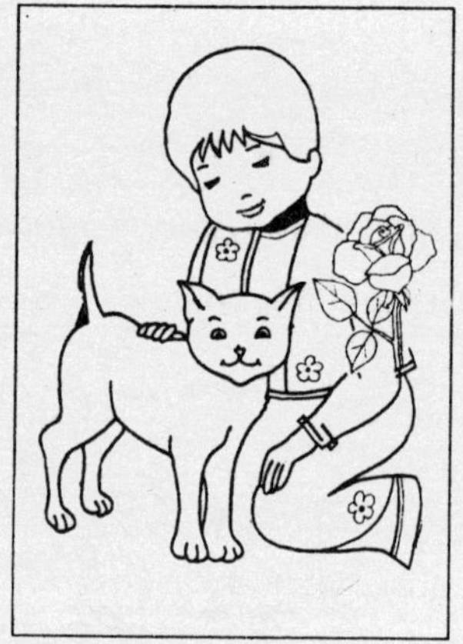

A child counts on his parents and grandparents for leadership, love and security. He also watches their parents instinct and patterns himself. This way a child develops his ability to cope.

What is the greatest gift to a child from his parents?

It is love which they want and express in countless ways, spontaneous expression of physical expression. Caregivers love creates an answering love in children.

Are both parents needed for a child's development?

It is preferable to have a child live with both parents as the child will then know both the sexes realistically and will be able to follow a marital relationship.

Does a boy need a friendly father?

Every father wants his son to achieve excellence in life. But if father is constantly criticizing, even in a friendly tone, the boy becomes uncomfortable inside.

Does a girl need a friendly father too?

Yes, friendly father plays a different but equally important part in the development of a girl. She gains confidence in herself as a girl and a woman from feeling his approval. She learns to enjoy the masculine qualities in her father while she is getting ready for her adult life. Her life is influenced by the kind of relationship she has with her father.

What if there is only one parent?

A child growing up with a caring single parent is better than a child whose mother and father neglect his needs because of their own unhappiness or circumstances. Children need love, give them that and they will flourish and blossom.

When is whining most common?

Whining is the pattern of excessive demandingness, specially during preschool days. Many children whine at only one parent, not both although some are equal opportunity whiners.

Why do some parents meet the excessive demands of their toddlers?

Parents believe that demanding something is the birthright of children. Not meeting the demand of children makes them feel guilty.

Do doctors make good parents?

No, not always. They always remain more concious and do not allow the child to grow normally. They will boil water for twenty minutes before giving to child and will not allow child to play on the ground fearing bacterial infection. As a result such children do not develop good immunity and fall sick off and on.

Why certain children do not leave their mothers even for a minute?

Such children are hyperactive and suffer from extreme separation anxiety. This requires a supportive environment. Try to involve someone else when you are playing with him. Introduce toys and let him play when you are around. Gradually make him feel more secure and don't be overprotective.

Should parents love a boy and a girl equally?

Start loving them uniquely, instead equally, because each gender has its own needs, likes and dislikes. You have to study each one, observe and then behave accordingly. This needs a lot of time and patience.

FOOD

What happens when a child tastes sugar for the first time?

The child is immediately attracted to the taste of sugar. This attraction is innate. Innate drive helped primitive man select safe foods avoiding bitter tasting substances which were often poisonous.

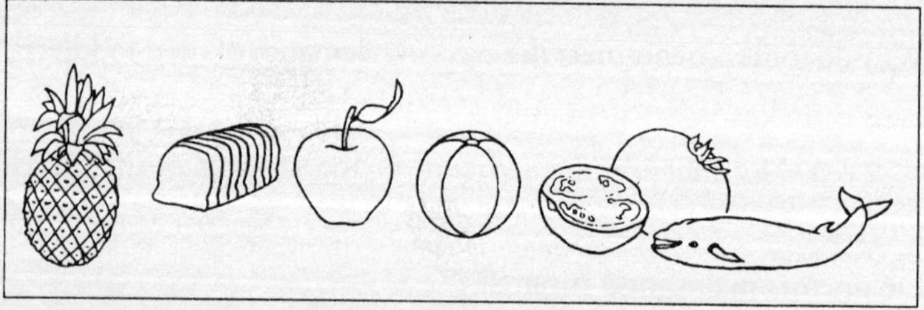

There is no conclusive evidence to prove that sugar has any effect on child's behaviour or learning. Still start giving your child a diet free of refined and artificial sugars too.

How to feed fruits to begin with?

Generally babies become used to cereals first, then vegetables and then fruits. Apple juice or stew is first given along with mashed ripe bananas. Increase one fruit at a time and the baby will learn to like each one.

Do children need high protein foods?

Once the baby is familiar with cereals, vegetables, fruits and kidney beans, soyabean preparations can be introduced. One need not to be a nonvegetarian in order to get sufficient proteins in one's diet.

When to give finger foods?

At the age of 7-8 months when the child can pick food up in his hands. They will not like spoon feeding if they are not permitted to feed themselves with their fingers. Babies love being offered pieces of food from their parents' plates.

How do teeth develop?

A baby gets his first tooth at about 7 month and around 1 year. He may have 4 to 6 sharp biting teeth. A baby does not get his first molars for grinding the food until about the 15th month.

What is the utility of an egg to a child?

Iron in egg yolk is poorly absorbed by a child's intestine. On the contrary it interferes in iron absorption from outside, unless

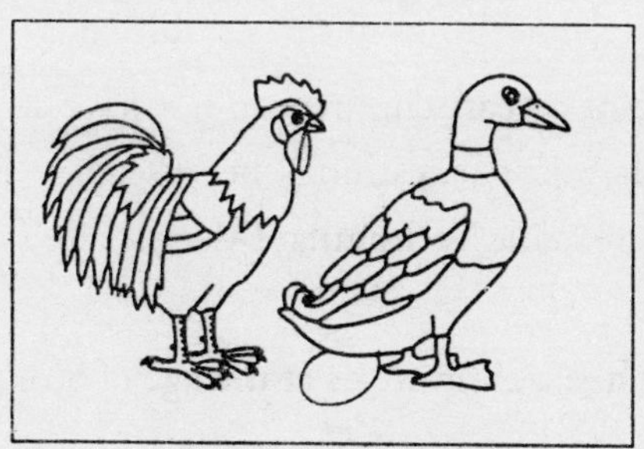

vitamin C is taken along with it. Egg yolk is a rich source of cholesterol. White portion of an egg is protein. You may consult doctor that how many eggs a week will be beneficial to child.

What foods are to be avoided?

- Sugary foods – Soft drinks and sweets promote cavities and spoil the baby's appetite.
- Nonvegetarian foods – A child on a vegetarian diet will have tremendous advantage throughout life avoiding heart diseases and bacterial infections.
- Tea/Coffee – Caffeine is found in colas, black tea and chocolates. Its stimulant effect is better avoided.
- Honey – It should not be given before 1 year because it may contain botulism spores which a child's intestines cannot kill.

Why do certain children stand and play at meals?

Actually a child is more keen in all other kinds of activities than food. He likes, climbing, handling the spoon, dropping something on the floor. Fooling around at meals is a sign of a child's growth.

STEALING

What about stealing things in early childhood?

Up to the age of 3 years children do not have any clear sense of belonging. They just take things because they like them. It is better not to redicule or humilate them. Parents should guide them.

What to do when a child steals at the age of 5 or more?

Deal with the child firmly. Do not allow him to lie. This is the time to think whether the child needs more affection and help. For that parents may take the help of a child guidance clinic.

SEPARATION

How does separation anxiety affect?

A baby of 6-8 months is likely to go in to depression if his caretaking mother is absent due to illness or is away on a tour. The baby looses his appetite and becomes unresponsive to known and unknown people. He lies down on his back rolling his head from side to side.

How does a separated child of 2–2½ years of age behave?

Separation from mother may not produce depression. The child may enjoy the company of the babysitter but when parents return in the evening the child rushes cling to them. He cries out if mother does not lift him. At bedtime the child will not leave his mother or father.

How does a child of 5-6 years of age behave if he is left at school?

A few children may resist being left at school. Caretaker has to stay in campus for a few days so that child may develop confidence.

PLAY

Can a hyperactive child play with toys?

Why not? Rather he should be provided with different types of colourful toys to attract him.

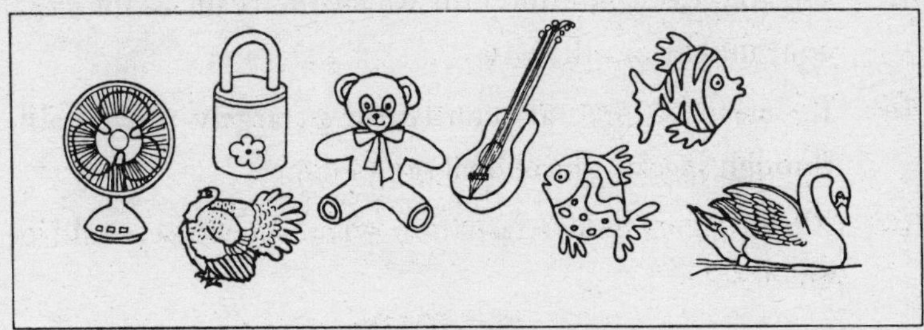

Why do many children like cars more?

Actually speaking a child of 1 year will be facinated by any moving object producing alarm, sound or light like cars, train and aeroplane.

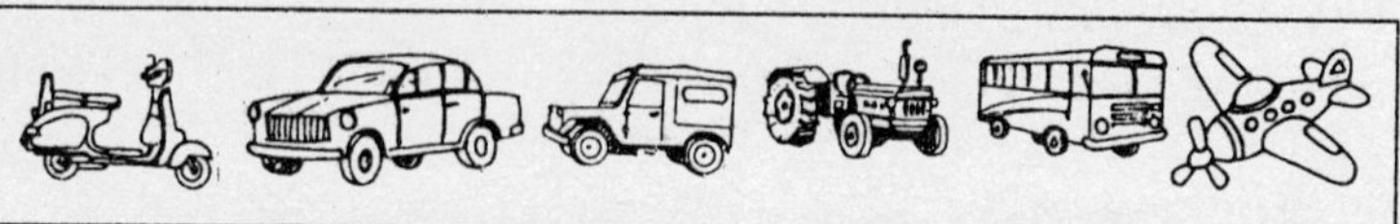

MENTAL RETARDATION

Who is a mentally retarded child?

A person is said to be mentally retarded when he is functioning much below the average level for his age atleast in two of the following areas

- Language skill
- Intellectual capacity
- Ability to take care of himself
- Social skill
- School work
- Vocational abilities

What are the causes of mental retardation?

(i) Organic cases are those in which the brain is abnormal congenitally or otherwise

(ii) Experiential mental retardation is largely preventable through special educational programmes.

(iii) Idiopathic mental retardation where no cause could be established.

HIV INFECTION

Can a HIV infected mother breast feed?

Infants born who are not infected at birth can get infected through breast feeding. HIV is commonly contained in the breast milk of HIV infected mother. So if the mother can maintain and sustain then she may put child on artificial feeds.

What about immunization in HIV infected infant?

Killed vaccine such as DPT Hepatitis-B vaccine should be given as schedule. Oral Polio Vaccine should not be given because of

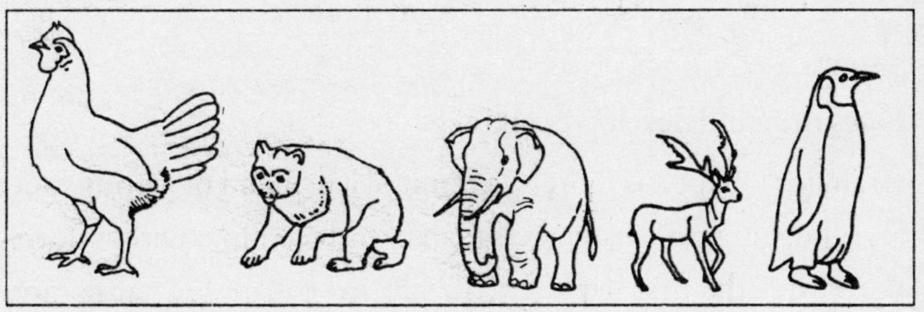

possibility of vaccine associated poliomyelitis. Inactivated polio vaccine is recommended. MMR vaccine and Measle vaccine should be given as per schedule.

TEETHING

When does the first tooth appear?

The first tooth erupts at about 6 months. Symptoms of teething include drooling and irregular chewing starting as early as 4 months. Time of appearance of teeth may vary but the sequence remains the same. The two lower central incisors are first to appear. Two upper central incisors usually appear next, followed by four lateral incisors. These 8 teeth appear by the age of 1 year.

The first four molars are next in line. The crown of the tooth develops first. By the age of 3 years, 20 teeth appear.

When do permanent teeth appear?

By 6 years of age, permanent teeth start pushing up and the milk teeth start falling one by one, making space for permanent teeth.

Does fever develop during teething?

Actually viral and bacterial infections cause fever. Low grade fever develops due to inflammation of gums. It may be due to the infant putting many things in the mouth.

Eardrum and teeth share a common nerve so pain in ear may also be felt.

Does the child develop crankiness?

Crankiness happens more as a result of a demand of getting more love, hugging from caretakers than of real teething. Discomfort is more with the first teeth. Eventually, the molar will cause more discomfort due to its large size.

During the crawling stage the child may pick up things, put them in his mouth and get infection which leads to his being unwell and cranky.

Why does a child get diarrhoea during teething?

While cutting the first teeth, most of the children develop diarrhoea. During this period the child swallows a lot of saliva. Putting every thing in his mouth to get relief from pain may further result in infection and diarrhoea.

How to take care of teeth?

Rub honey on the gums with your clean fingers. Clean fingers will remove any plaque/bacteria. Avoid fluoride tooth paste with infants under the age of 2 years because they may swallow it.

A NAUGHTY CHILD

How does a child become naughty at the age of 1 year?

At the age of 1 year and above, the child starts discovering his newly acquired physical skills. He starts pushing furniture, and feeding himself. He likes to explore his surroundings.

Your child's first step is the stepping stone to freedom. He feels excited as he puts his foot forward and sees the excitement he generates all around him.

What precautions should parents take?

At this stage try and remove breakable items from within the child's reach. Every minute he would like to explore new things so –

- Keep cupboards properly locked.
- Do not leave your child all alone in the bathroom.
- Put potentially dangerous items such as medicines, sharp objects, pointed kitchen knives and forks, hot drinks, etc., out of the child's reach.

Why do children always want to go out of the house?

Between the age of 1 to 2 years a child starts manifesting social behaviour and becomes comfortable with strangers. He eagerly looks for an opportunity to go out to see different objects, animals and meet people.

In the garden some day, he will tug free of your hand and before you can stop him, he will be racing into the play ground. But the next day he may not leave you and remain in your lap.

These growing months will be full of surprises.

What to do when two children start fighting?

You will notice that children will push, snatch things and even hit each other. Do not get alarmed or perturbed, neither jump to protect the child. He will learn to fend for himself. His being alone will develop confidence in him and a positive sense of himself.

CHILD TELLING TALES

When does a child start telling tales?

Preschool children start learning how to separate fantasy from reality but they still do not know what the actual truth is. The child is still swayed by forgetfulness, wishful thinking and imagination. He may forget where he has kept his things. Children have very short memory. So on many occasions the child may not remember the truth.

Do children lie?

Your preschool child may realise that his misdeed will disappoint you. So instead of facing your displeasure he may lie. Also creating stories may make him feel important. He may exaggerate the facts.

What is the best way to teach him truthfulness?

The best way to teach honesty is to be honest. Children learn from parents. You should try to set a good example. Try to keep your word.

Should parents blame the child?

If you blame your child for lying, he may just go on denying it to avoid disappointing you. You should talk to him to reassure him. If he has eaten chocolate secretly then instead of scolding, you may offer him chocolate yourself; or you should try to make him understand that chocolates can cause painful cavities in his teeth.

Do not call your child a 'lier', although you should make it clear that you do not like lies. Say it gently but firmly.

SELF-ESTEEM

How to nurture self-esteem in children?

Children should have a good feeling about themselves. Such children handle conflicts easily. For this to happen, parents should communicate with the child about his choices, hopes and dreams.

Should children be allowed to express their emotions?

You should encourage your child to express his feelings. For that they need your support. Whatever they may express, do not label them as stupid or crazy. Children are very sensitive to parents' words. Rather always give a positive and accurate feedback to him.

Should parents listen to children?

Invite your child to discuss. Active listening builds self-esteem. Do not dictate them but solve their problem. Be like a friend to your child. Establish the best opportunity to develop strong moral and spiritual values in him.

What type of environment should parents develop?

A child whose parents always go on fighting and arguing, may become depressed and withdrawn. His self-esteem will be low. Make your house a model haven for child.

Should parents have some fun time with children?

Children like laughing parents. Laugh at jokes and mistakes too. Go out on a picnic, take a family vacation and spend your weekends with your children.

SHARING

What is expected from children?

Up to 4-5 years, children may laugh and play together but they do not share their toys. Only at 6-8 years do they learn to share.

Should parents show generosity?

If you are generous, your child will like to copy you. You should give your child the opportunity to mix with people and see the world for himself. Teach him to think about friends and members of the family. You could be involved in charitable activity too. Try not to resort to punishment in case he gives away things which he is not supposed to. Explain the joys of correct sharing and carying to him.

SIBLING RIVALRY

Do siblings develop jealousy?

Most of us have had sibling rivalry. Although siblings are proud of each other, they seldom express it.

Parents should not encourage jealousy. They should make their children understand that one may be good in one thing and another may be better in something else. A parent should not favour anyone outright. You should support both of them.

Should parents do compare their children?

It is but natural for parents to notice that one of their children is more co-operative or better behaved than other. But comparing siblings does not encourage better behaviour. It only intensifies jealousy and envy.

What should be the parents' role when the children fight?

When it comes to a fight among siblings it is best not to take sides. Do not put too much focus in trying to find out who started the fight or who is at fault. Let them work out their differences. Get involved in serious matters only and separate the children until they are calm. The more you stay out of minor fights, the sooner they will learn to settle their differences.

Is sibling rivalry always harmful?

Some effects of sibling conflict may even prove helpful in the long run. Children learn to cope with disagreements and disputes. They learn to value another person's perspective and they learn to compromise and negotiate. They learn to control aggressive impulses. They also learn about sharing and co-operation.

Does a younger sibling develop social skills better?

Yes, as a child reaches the age of 3 years he becomes aware of how his elder brothers have been enriched with the addition of friends. He comes to know that friends provide new opportunities, interactions and experiences. So it is likely that he will make friends more easily than his elder sibling.

How children squable?

Ties with siblings are often the strongest lifelong relationship people have.

- Most young children spend a certain amount of time bickering and fighting.
- During preschool years they show little affection for each other and squable off and on.
- In middle childhood the amount of warmth and companionship may increase.
- During teenage they may turn away from family and develop friendship.
- If age difference between two siblings is more, older kid may feel burdened by having to spend time with a much younger one.

How should an elder child behave when a new baby arrives in house?

Encourage an elder one to attend and play with the new arrival. Older sibling will take pride in speaking slowly but clearly to a new baby so that he can learn the language. The younger baby , with the older siblings help, will develop certain milestones earlier.

How does the family affect siblings' behaviour?

Sibling rivalry is least likely to occur where –

- Parents do not fight and find solutions respectfully.
- Where physical aggression and name-calling is not acceptable.
- Family members enjoy picnics, parties and ceremonies.

STRAY FACTS

Why do certain children bite a lot?

They learn this to be a means of drawing attention to themselves. Parents have to give quality time to their child so that he does not feel neglected. Give proper time in a proper way and do not scold the child. Stop explaining his behaviour in front of others.

What about the magic of touch?

The sense of touch is a powerful and highly sensitive form of communication. Special bonding is developed unknowingly when a mother cuddles her baby.

How does massaging of a baby help?

Massage helps in reducing the heart rate, lowering blood pressure, increasing blood circulation and lymph flow. It relaxes tense muscles. It increases endorphins which are a baby's natural pain killers.

What about the children who are nail nibblers?

Children start biting nails mostly at the age of 10. Even at the age of 5 children may pick up this habit seeing seniors biting their nails. Nail biting is also one of the 'tensional outlet'. Some children chew their nails when they are under special stress.

Is sibling rivalry natural?

Yes sibling rivalry is natural and normal where there are brothers and sisters to share their parents' love. Sometimes jealousy in interests can result in quarelling. It deprives the children of companionship.

Are teenagers more violent?

Teenagers are the usual targets of efforts to prevent violence and deliquency but science has discovered that human viciousness actually peaks in toddlers. We are lucky in one respect that a two year old child cannot do much harm. Still if you don't help the worst cases at this early stage, you might never be able to help them at all.

Is physical aggression a disease?

Physical aggression is not an illness one catches. It is a natural behaviour that one learns to control.

Do children like music?

Music has a tranquilising effect. Children like 'lullabies' and rhymes

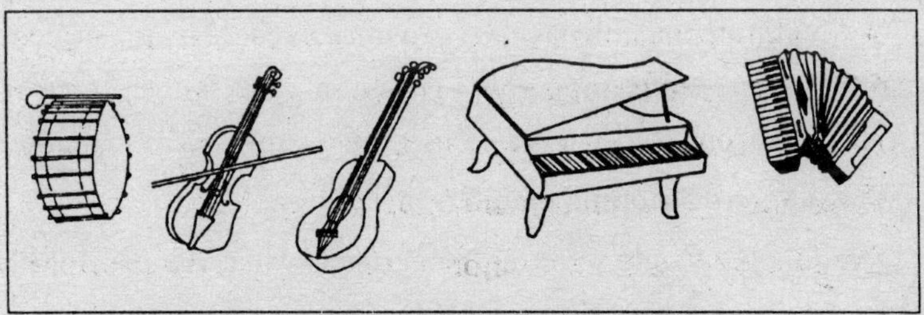

while adults prefer classical music and spiritual music in the morning. Good music is a tonic.

When does dissatisfaction in children start?

Dissatisfaction and decline begin to take root in childhood. Children are attracted to fancy toys and junk food. They may become obese and dull. The crippling burden of homework leaves them with little time to play and enjoy the bounties of nature.

How shyness affects children?

These are the kids the teachers tend to ignore because they do not make any demands, the ones you might see on the playground, hovering at the edge of the crowd, as if they wish to join in but are not sure how to do it. They are easy pickings for the classroom bully. They are painfully aware they do not fit in and are unable to face heart breaking loneliness. The shy child is rejected from his peer group.

What are the risk factors of shyness?

Shy kids have a greater risk for depression in adulthood and can be slow to take major life steps like starting careers and families.

What is the biology of child anxiety?

Infants and toddlers with higher heart rates at rest or greater activity in the right fronted part of their brains that handle negative emotions – ending up looking more socially anxious as preschoolers. An environmental link has also been uncovered. Having one good friend or caretaker may give protection against these factors. Children prone to shyness are raised by overprotective parents.

What about developing manners in children?

Decades ago people were more courteous when the pace of life was slower and people were not in a race to compete. But now many parents seem to feel that it is too old fashioned to care about manners. They feel that children should be allowed to develop naturally. Good manners come naturally. Some still feels that children are to be taught manners.

Why does a child's habit of biting disappear by the age of 3 years?

Children of 1-3 years cannot express their frustration or desire in words and they often retort biting. But after the age of 3, a child has learned to use words to express his desires instead of biting.

Who are hyperactive children?

Diagnosis is based solely on a child's behaviour. Boys are commonly affected by it. The child is very active with a short span of attention. He may also have a hot temper and be emotionally immature. These children have learning disabilities. Doctor should be consulted.

Can a child develop dandruff?

Dandruff develops as small whitish scales of skin which come loose on combing. There may be itching. In severe cases skin and hair becomes greasy with patches of reddish skin. Oozed fluid become hard with yellow crusts. Shampoo kills the microorganism. Excessive shampooing or massaging may over stimulate making the condition worse. Some medicated antidandruff shampoos are available in the market.

What is childhood diabetes?

Insufficient insulin production of pancreas results in childhood diabetes. Blood sugar level rises making the child more thirsty. He drinks excessively and passes a lot of urine. Child may loose weight and feel unwell. Only injection of insulin helps in such cases.

Section Two

Immunisation

Dr. Abhitabh

How are diseases transmitted?

Diseases may be transmitted from reservoir or source of infection to a suceptible individual in many different ways

(i) Direct transmission

- Direct contact
- Droplet infection
- Contact with soil
- Inoculation into skin

(ii) Indirect transmission

- Vehicle borne
- Vector borne
- Air borne
- Fomite borne

How are diseases spread by direct contact?

Disease can spread by touching, kissing or sexual intercourse. Such Diseases include STD, AIDS, leprosy, skin and eye infections.

What are droplet infections?

This is a direct projection of a spray of droplet of saliva and naso-pharyngeal secretions during coughing or sneezing. The droplet spread is usually limited to a distance of 30-60 cm. Such diseases include eruptive fevers, common cold, diphtheria, whooping cough, tuberculosis and meningitis.

What is immunisation?

It is one of the most effective means of preventing infectious diseases in children. Over 11 antigens are used today for routine immunisation of infants and children.

What are live vaccines?

Live vaccines include BCG, measles, oral polio prepared from live organisms. Live vaccines are more potent immunizing agent than killed vaccines. Live vaccines must be properly stored to retain effectiveness. Serious failures to measles and polio immunisation have resulted due to faulty refrigeration.

What are killed vaccines?

These are organisms killed by heat or chemicals when infected into the body stimulating active immunity. These are safe but less effective. Efficacy of 3 doses of pertussis is 50% only and after 12 years this reduces to zero. Killed vaccines are given intramuscularly.

Can vaccines be combined?

Yes, the aim of a combined vaccine is to simplify administration and to reduce cost. Following are some of vaccines available.

- DPT (Diphtheri-Pertussis-Tetanus)
- DT (Diptheria-tetanus)
- DP (Diphtheria-Pertussis)
- DPT and typhoid vaccine
- MMR (Measles, mumps and rubella)
- DPTP (DPT + inactivated polio)

What is a cold chain?

A cold chain is a system of storage and transport of vaccines at low temperature from the production site to actual vaccination site.

Among these vaccines polio is the most sensitive to heat, requiring the storage of minus 20 degree C. Vaccines which must be stored in freezer are polio, measles and BCG. Vaccines which are to kept in refrigerator but not in the freezer include typhoid, DPT, and tetanus toxoid.

Vaccines must be protected from sunlight and antibiotics.

Which diseases require isolation?

Diseases which require isolation and the period of separation required of the infected person from others to prevent spread of communicable diseases are given below.

What is the recommended period of isolation?

Disease	Duration of Isolation
Chicken pox	Until all lesions are crusted. 6 days after onset of rash
Measles	From the onset of catarrhal stage to 3rd day of rash
Diphtheria	For 48 hours after patient becomes negative
Hepatitis A	3 weeks
Influenza	3 days after onset of disease
Polio	6 weeks pediatrics; 2 weeks adult
Tuberculosis Sputum +	Until 3 weeks of effective chemotherapy
Mumps	Until swelling subsides
Pertussis	4 weeks
Pharyngitis	6 hours of effective antibiotics

What is the revised National Immunisation Programme of India?

Beneficiaries	Age	Vaccine
Infants	At birth	BCG, OPV
	6 weeks	DPT, OPV
	10 weeks	DPT, OPV
	14 weeks	DPT, OPV
	9 months	Measles
Children	15-18 months	MMR Ist booster dose of DPI, OPV
	4½-5 years	DT
	10 years	TT
	15 years	TT
Pregnant women	16-36 weeks	TT two doses 4 weeks apart

What is DTP?

DTP is dephtheria + tetanus + pertussis. It is given to the baby at the ages of 6, 10 and 14 weeks. Booster dose may be given around 15-18 weeks. Crocin drops may be given before the vaccine so that the baby does not develop fever. It is common for a small, firm lump or knot to form in the thigh or the arm where the injection has been given.

What about polio vaccine?

This oral vaccine is given at birth, 6th, 10th, 14th week and at 15 months. When oral vaccine is used some live polio virus comes out in feces and caregiver may get viral infection if he is susceptible.

How does MMR reacts?

It contains vaccine against measles, mumps and rubella. This triple vaccine contains live weakened viruses. Reaction to measles vaccine develops after a week resembling measles. One in 10 children will develop a fever higher than 103^0F.

Is chicken pox vaccine available?

It is now recommended for children between 1 to 13 years who have not already had chicken pox.

Can a Hepatitis B vaccine be given?

It is a series of 3 shots recommended to all children. Older children and adults may also be given.

Common Diseases Affecting Children

Dr. Abhishek Gupta

DIARRHOEA

What is the importance of diarrhoea?

Acute diarrhoeal disease is one of the major causes of morbidity and mortality in India. Up to the age of 5 every child suffers from at least 2 episodes of diarrhoea. 10% of these are likely to develop dehydration.

What is diarrhoea?

Diarrhoea may be defined as passing of 3 or more loose motions or watery stools in a day. Frequent passing of normal stool is not diarrhoea.

What are the common causes of diarrhoea?

Acute diarrhoea with or without nausea and vomiting may occur due to variety of causes. Rota virus is more frequent in children. Other causes include bacterial infection, amoebiasis, giardiasis etc. As infants put every thing in their mouths they catch infection more easily.

What happens during diarrhoea?

There is a loss of a large amount of water and salts from the body. Water and electrolytes are also lost through vomit, sweat, urine and fast breathing.

Dehydration occurs faster in infants and young children in hot climate, specially when the patient has a temperature.

What are the signs of dehydration?

Common signs are

- Restlessness or irritability

- Lethargy
- Sunken eyes
- Pinched skin returns slowly to normal.
- Thirst and the patient drinks eagerly

How to prevent dehydration?

Simple diarrhoea with no obvious dehydration can be treated by mothers at home with lemon water, butter milk, rice water (kanji), dal soup, green coconut water, diluted milk, weak tea and breast milk.

What are the rules of home treatment?

- If the child is breast fed, try to give breast milk more often. If the child is not breast fed, then increase the normal milk feed with diluted milk.
- A child under 2 years of age should be given 50-100 ml of fluid after each loose stool and older children should receive twice the amount. Adults may take as much as they want.
- All children above 6 months should be given easily digestable solid food such as boiled rice, porridge, soups, etc. No child should be starved.
- If the child does not improve within 12-18 hours, ORS may be given.

What is the composition of ORS?

Oral Rehydration Salt contains

Ingredients	Amount
Glucose	20.0 grams
Sodium chloride	3.5 grams
Sodium bicarbonate	2.5 grams
Potassium chloride	1.5 grams

ORS solution should be made fresh every day and the left over solution must be discarded.

How does one assess dehydration?

No exact formula can be given for assessing dehydration. It requires a careful evaluation of history and physical examination.

Assessment of dehydration

Signs and Symptoms	Mild dehydration	Moderate dehydration	Severe dehydration
• General condition	• Thirsty, alert, restless	• Thirsty, restless irritable on touch	• Drowsy, limp sweaty, cyanotic limbs
• Radial Pulse	• Normal rate and volume	• Rapid and weak	• Rapid, feeble or may not be palpable.
• Respiration	• Normal	• Rapid and weak	• Deep and rapid
• Ant. Fontanella	• Normal	• Sunken	• Very Sunken
• Blood pressure	• Normal	• Low	• May be not recordable
• Skin elasticity	• Pinch retracts	• Pinch retracts slowly	• Retracts very slowly > 2 seconds
• Eye	• Normal	• Sunken	• Deeply sunken
• Mucous membrane	• Moist	• Dry	• Very dry
• Urine flow	• Normal	• Dark and reduced	• Not passing urine
• % body wt. loss	• 4-5%	• 6-9%	• 10% or more
• Estimated fluid deficit	• 40-50 ml/ kg	• 60-90 ml/kg	• 100-100 ml/kg

What to do during rehydration therapy?

- Breast fed infants – After the first 4 hours of rehydration therapy breast feeding should be started and thereafter continued as often as the infant desires, in addition to continuing ORS solution.
- Non breast, infant – After 4 hours of rehydration therapy plain water should be given equal to half the volume of ORS solution already taken by the infant.
- Older children – May be given as much water as they want.

What is a maintenance therapy?

After the initial fluid and electrolyte deficit has been corrected, it is important to replace the ongoing losses of fluid and electrolytes that are associated with continuing diarrhoea. This is known as maintenance therapy. It can be met in the following ways.

- Breast fed infants – Breast feeding should be allowed as often as the infant desires, in addition to the required volume of ORS solution.
- Non breast fed infants – Milk consumed by the infant can be restarted but should be diluted with equal amount of clean water until diarrhoea stops. It should be given along with ORS.

What to do in case of vomiting occuring after ORS?

Vomiting may be there during the first hour or two after ORS, but it does not prevent successful oral rehydration. To reduce vomiting give ORS slowly, in sips at short intervals. But when severe vomiting occurs then intravenous therapy should be used.

When should ORS to be given through nasogastric tube?

A bay who cannot drink due to fatigue or drowsiness but are not in shock a nasogastric tube can be used to give ORS solutions.

What solutions are available for intravenous infusion?

A number of solutions are available.

- Ringer's solution – It is the best commerciably available solution. It provides sufficient sodium, potassium and lactate yielding bicarbonate for correction of acidosis. It can be given to all age groups for dehydration of all causes.
- Normal saline – It is easily available but will not correct acidosis and will not replace potassium losses.

Which is the unsuitable solution?

Plain glucose and dextrose solutions are not to be used as they provide only water and sugar. It does not contain electrolyte so electrolyte losses are not corrected, neither does it correct acidosis.

PERSISTENT DIARRHOEA

What is persistent diarrhoea?

It is a diarrhoea with or without blood which begins acutely and lasts for 14 days or longer.

How to manage severe persistent diarrhoea?

ORS solution is effective for most children with persistent diarrhoea. When glucose absorption is impaired then ORS solution is not effective. In such cases when ORS is given their thirst and stool quantity increases markedly. Signs of dehydration worsen. Stool examination may show large amount of unabsorbed glucose. These children require I.V. rehydration. Antibiotics are not effective unless diarrhoea is with blood.

How should an infant aged under 4 months be fed?

- One should encourage exclusive breast feeding.

- If child is not breast feeding give a breast milk substitute which is low in lactose such as yoghurt. Use spoon or cup as a feeding bottle should not be used for this.

How to feed a child older than 5 months in persistent diarrhoea?

Once diarrhoea is controlled, the child may be given food 6 times a day to gain 100 calories/kg/day. Many children will eat poorly.

What about weight loss during diarrhoea?

Many children will loose weight for 1-2 days and then steadily gain weight when infection subsides after 7 days. Weight gain will start.

CHRONIC DIARRHOEA

What should be the feeding pattern in case of chronic diarrhoea?

- If still breast feeding, give more frequent and longer feeds.
- If taking animal milk, start giving yoghurt.
- Give other foods to ensure an adequate calorie intake.

What should be the supplementary micronutrient?

One should supplement

- Folate 50 micrograms
- Zinc 10 mg
- Iron 10 mg
- Vitamin A, 400 microgram
- Copper 1 mg
- Magnesium 60 mg at least.

DYSENTERY

How does one detect dysentery?

Dysentery is diarrhoea with loose frequent stools with blood. Most episodes are due to shigella and nearly all need antibiotics.

What are the features of bacillary dysentery?

The characteristic features are sudden fever followed by spasmodic pain in abdomen and frequent loose stools. There will be tenesmus, i.e. acute rectal discomfort. Later on there may be dysentric feaces consisting of blood, mucus and fecal matter mixed intimately.

What should be the treatment?

Children with severe malnutrition below 2 months should be admitted in hospital.

Give an oral antibiotic for 5 days to which strains of shigella are locally sensitive. Antibiotics may be ampicillin and nalidixic acid.

What are the signs of improvement?

Following are the signs of improvement

- Disappearance of fever
- Less blood in stool
- Passage of fewer stools
- Improvement of appetite
- Child becoming physically active.

Should one give symptomatic relief?

Never give drugs for symptomatic relief of abdominal pain and rectal pain, or to reduce the frequency of stools. All this may mask the under current severity of illness.

What should be the nutritional management?

- Breast feeding should be continued throughout the period of illness. Children between 4-6 months should get normal food, whatever they were consuming. To compensate loss of potassium, banana, coconut water and green leafy vegetables may be given.

AMOEBIC DYSENTERY

It is caused by entamoeba histolytica by way of oral route. The infection is generally spread by way of contaminated food and water. The cyst wall is dissolved in alkalive reaction of small intestine liberating the tropozoites or vegetative forms directly responsible for damage of intestinal mucosa.

What is its characteristic features?

There are frequent loose or even watery offensive stools containing mucosal blood. There will be griping abdominal pain over lower abdomen near around umbilicus. Child looks dull and fatigued.

Who are the asymptomatic carriers?

Cooks or servants who do not present any specific complaint but are generally detected as cyst passers on routine stool examination. These people are the source of spreading the disease. Course of metronidazole helps.

FEVER

The normal temperature of the body is 98.4^{0}F or 37^{0}C. In case of children the temperature should not be allowed to go beyond 103^{0}F. High fever may cause irritation of brain meninges resulting in convulsions. It may result in serious complications.

How does one change values of centrigrade into farenheit?

With the help of following table you can interchange the values

Centigrade	Farenheit	Centigrade	Farenheit	Centigrade	Frenheit
36.5	97.7	38.4	101.1	39.7	103.5
36.8	98.2	38.6	101.5	40.0	104.0
37.2	98.4	38.8	101.8	40.2	104.4
37.4	99.0	38.9	102.0	40.4	104.7
37.6	99.7	39.0	102.2	40.7	105.4
37.8	100.2	39.2	102.6	41.0	105.5
38.0	100.4	39.5	103.1	41.0	106.0

What is a thermometre?

It is an instrument, containing mercury, which is used to measure the temperature of a body. High temperature alters the volume of the mercury. The temperature is a degree of warmth or coldness of a substance. The bulb of a temperature is filled with mercury because mercury acquires the body temperature easily and quickly. It does not wet the glass. Constriction prevents mercury from falling back after the thermometre has been taken out of the human body. There is an arrow in red indicating the normal level of 98.4^{0}F. Every degree is subdivided into five parts, each representing 0.2^{0}F.

What is the procedure of taking temperature by mouth?

If the patient has had a cold or hot drink, wait for 15 minutes before checking the temperature.

- Hold the thermometre by its tip and shake it down by a sharp movement of the wrist until the mercury column drops below 37^{0}C.
- Place the bulb end under the patient's tongue. Be careful to

see that child does not break it. A child usually understands the procedure after the age of 7-8 years. After the thermometre has been placed under the tongue, the child should close his mouth.

- Leave the thermometre for 2 minutes and read after taking it out.

What is the procedure of an oral thermometre to record temperature in axilla and groin?

- Wipe the axilla or groin so that it dries up.
- For axillary temperature place the thermometer in the armpit of the child and bring the arm down so that it touches the side of the chest with elbow bent and the forearm placed across the abdomen.
- Leave the thermometre for 2 minutes. After that read the figure. Similarly thermometer can be placed in the groin.

How to record rectal temperature?

- Use rectal thermometre having globular bulb.
- Place the infant on its abdomen, preferably on the lap of mother. Also keep a piece of cloth handy for use in case he passes stool.
- Moisten a cotton swab with oil or other lubricant and lubricate the bulb end of the thermometre.
- Gently insert the bulb into the anus for about 3 cm. Do not use force because you may pierce the wall of the rectum.
- Leave the thermometre for 2 minutes. Normal rectal temperature is 37.5°C (99.6°F) or one degree higher than oral temperature.

How temperature helps in diagnosis?

Observation	Possible Problem
Cool moist skin	Shock, bleeding, heat exhaution
Cool dry skin	Exposure to cold
Cool clammy skin	Shock
Hot dry skin	High fever, heat stroke
Hot moist skin	Infection

MEASLES

What type of symptoms does one get in measles?

Measles is a highly contagious viral disease with serious complications. It generally does not develop in a child before 3 months of age. After 1-2 weeks of incubation the disease presents itself with cough, mild conjunctivitis, nasal discharge and fever.

Small grey-white lesions known as koplick's spots appear on the posterior buccal mucosa. Fine rashes develop over ears and spreads to become generalised and blotchy. Rashes last only for 4 days. The rash may lead to skin desquamation.

What are its prominent features?

Commonest features are

- Fever
- Generalized minute rashes
- Cough/running nose/red eyes

What can be the complication?

- Child may develop inability to drink or breast feed.

- Vomits everything.
- Convulsions.
- Lethargy.

Child may develop pus discharge from ear, diarrhoea or pneumonia.

How to manage a case of measle?

The role of antibiotics is to prevent chest infection. If temperature is more than 102^{0}F give paracetamol. But if fever continues for 3-4 days it is indicative of secondary infection and sponging with cold water, specially of forehead, palms and soles, will help. Take off the clothes of the child.

SEPTICAEMIA

If a child has acute fever with severe illness but does not have any obvious cause then septicaemia may be suspected. Wherever meningococcal disease is common, meningococcal septicaemia may be considered.

What are the clinical features of septicaemia?

The following are its clinical features

- Fever with no obivious focus of infection.
- Blood film for M.P. to be prepared to rule out malaria.
- See for stiff neck to rule out meningitis.
- Unable to breast feed, convulsions, lethargy and vomiting.

How to manage such cases?

- Consult the doctor.
- Child will require hospital care and antibiotics.
- Don't allow fever above 102^{0}F. Complications of

septicaemia includes shock dehydration, pneumonia and coma.

TYPHOID FEVER

One should suspect typhoid fever if child has vomiting, pain, diarrhoea/constipation and fever of more than 7 days and when malaria has been rule out.

What are its diagnostic features?

- Rise of fever in the evening.
- Fever never becomes normal.
- Relative slowing of pulse.
- Inability to drink or breast feed, leathargy, vomiting.

How to manage it?

Chloromycetin/ciprobid suspension should be used. Fluid bland diet will help. Fluids have to be maintained.

MASTOIDITIS

This is a bacterial infection of the mastoid cell behind the ear. Without treatment it may lead to meningitis and brain abscess.

What are its clinical signs?

It includes

- High fever.
- Pain and swelling behind ear.

How to manage it?

Suitable antibiotic in appropriate dose should be given otherwise surgical incision may be required. In complicated cases meningitis may develop.

ACUTE OTITIS MEDIA

This is an inflammation of the middle ear cavity behind the ear drum of less than 2 weeks. Fluid accumulates and causes pain due to increase of pressure in the cavity. When the eardum ruptures, pus discharges from the ear. It can be confirmed with the help of otoscopy.

How you will diagnose it?

This is based on a history of ear pain or pus draining from the ear. On otoscopy eardrum will be red, inflammed and immobile.

How you will treat it?

- Give suitable antibiotic.
- Tell the mother not to put anything in the ear.
- If pus is there the mother should dry the ear by wicking. The mother should clean the ear at least thrice a day.

COLIC

This is the most common cause of recurrent abdominal pain in infancy. The attacks come in paroxysms and is accompanied with severe crying.

What is aerophagy?

It is the excessive wind in gastronitestinal tract due to prolonged sucking, more so when the breast is empty. Inadequate burping may also cause it.

What are the symptoms of 'evening colic'?

It is characterized by paroxysms of abdominal pain lasting a few minutes at a time and occuring usually in the late evening. During pain, face is often flushed. Legs are drawn up over abdomen and feet are cold and hands become clenched. When the infant is exhausted attack dies down or passes flatus or stools.

Can cow's milk allergy be a cause for this?

This may be the cause only in a few cases . There may be vomiting watery diarrhoea, rhinitis and failure to grow. Withdrawl of cow's milk is followed by disappearance of the manifestations.

Can intestinal worms cause colicky pain?

Yes, intestinal infestation with L. giardia, E. histolytica, hook worm, trichuris trichura constitute by far the most frequent cause of recurrent abdominal pain. There will be change in appetite and failure to gain weight. Each and every child with recurrent abdominal pain must have at least 3 consecutive meticulous stool check ups.

Can there be psychogenic pain in the abdomen?

In a few cases abdominal pain may simply be a sort of attention seeking device. Child comes to know that parents bother only when his abdomen is paining.

What do you understand by abdominal epilepsy?

It is characterised by recurrent but sudden attacks of abdominal pain lasting for a few minutes and followed by sleep.

Can constipation lead to abdominal pain?

Yes, excessive drying of feaces leading to impaction and partial intestinal obstruction may be responsible for recurrent abdominal pain.

CHICKEN POX

It is an acute highly infectious disease caused by varicella zoster. Source of infection is usually a case of chicken pox.

How is it transmitted?

It is transmitted from person to person by droplet infection and by droplet neuclei. Most patients are infected by 'face to face' contact. Portal of entry of virus is respiratory tract. Virus can cross the placental barrier and infect the fetus. Incubation period is 14-16 days.

What are its clinical features?

(i) Preeruptive stage – In children onset is sudden with mild or moderate fever. Rarely will there be high fever. Rashes will be wide spread. There will be pain in the back. It takes 2-3 days before the rash develops.

(ii) Eruptive stage – In children rash may be the first sign along with fever.

What type of rashes develop?

Rashes appear symmetrically. On trunk these are abundant then they come on the face, arms and legs. Mucosa is generally involved. Axilla may be affected.

The rash advances quickly through the stage of macule, papule, vesicle and scab. These are superficial in nature. Scabbing begins within 4 to 7 days of the rash appearing.

All forms of rashes will appear at one point of time.

Mortality is less than 1% in uncomplicated cases.

How will you manage a case of chicken pox?

- Isolation.
- Applying talcum powder over body to avoid itching.
- Antibiotic is needed to avoid secondary infection.

MUMPS

This is a virus disease. Virus can be isolated from saliva. Period of communicability is 4-6 days before the onset of symptoms. It is the main cause of parotitis in children between 5-15 years. No age is exempt and no previous immunity works.

Disease spreads by droplet infection and by direct contact. Incubation period is 2 to 3 weeks.

What are its clinical features?

30% patients may not show any symptoms. Others will have pain and swelling of cheeks (parotid gland). A child complains of ear-pain. On opening the mouth the pain increases. Fever and headache may last for 3-5 days.

What are its complications?

Complications are frequent but not serious. There may be inflammation of testes, pancreas and heart muscle.

How can the disease be controlled?

It is difficult to control because the disease is infectious. However once diagnosed, cases should be isolated till the manifestations subside. One should disinfect the clothes. Antibiotics check complication. For pain, crocin syrup may be given.

DIPHTHERIA

It is an acutely infectious disease. Source of infection is a case or carrier. Mild or silent cases may not show any symptoms. Infective material is nasopharyngeal secretions, contaminated fomites and possibly infected dust.

Incubation period is 2-6 days.

What are its clinical features?

Patients with pharyngotonsillar diphtheria have a sore throat, difficulty in swallowing and low grade fever. Examination of the throat may show only mild erythema, localised exudate or a membrane. Membrane may be localised. If you remove these blue-white membrane there may develop bleeding.

How case of diphtheria can be managed?

- Isolation.
- When diphtheria is suspected diphtheria antitoxin should be given without delay 1.M or I.V. ranging 10,000 to 80,000 units or more.
- Carriers should be given 10 days course of erythromycin.
- Non-immunised close contact may be given 1000-2000 units of diphtheria antitoxin.

WHOOPING COUGH

This is an acutely infectious disease of young children caused by B-pertussis. There is insidious onset with mild fever and an irritating cough, gradually becoming paroxysmal with loud crowing inspiration. Causative agent is B. Pertussis. Source of infection is a case of pertussis. The bacilli occur abundantly in nasopharyngeal and bronchial secretion. Whooping cough is most infectious during the catarrhal stage. Infective period is 1-3 weeks after exposure.

It is primarily a disease of infants and preschool children. Incubation period is 7-14 days.

What is the clinical course of the disease?

It has 3 stages

(i) Catarrhal stage – lasting for about 10 days.

(ii) Paroxysmal stage – lasting for 2-4 weeks.

(iii) Convalescent stage – lasting for 1-2 weeks. Illness lasts 6-8 weeks.

How to manage the disease?

Erythromycin is the drug of choice. A dose of 30-50 mg/kg of body weight in 4 divided doses of 10 days is recommended. Antibiotics do not reduce the frequency or severity of spasm nor do they shorten the illness. They are useful in controlling secondary bacterial infection.

COMMON COLD-COUGH

These are common, self-limited viral infections that require only supportive care – Antibiotics are not needed. Wheezing occurs in some children. Most episodes end within 7-14 days.

What are its clinical features?

Clinical features include –

- Cough.
- Nasal discharge.
- Mouth breathing.
- Fever.
- There will be no fast breathing.

How to manage?

- Relieve high fever with paracetamol.
- Clear secretions from the child's nose before feeds.
- Normal saline nasal drops may be put after consulting the doctor.

OPHTHALIMIA NEONATORUM

This is also known as neonatal conjunctivitis. It is a severe purulent conjunctivitis in less than 1 month old infants. If not treated well this may lead to blindness. Causative organism is gonococcal infection acquired during the process of birth.

How can you treat it?

Kanamycin 25 mg/kg to a maximum of 75 mg in a single dose IM dose is effective. As a local treatment clean the newborn's eyes with 0.9% saline or clean water. Wipe from the inside to the outside using a clean swab for each eye. Wash your hands before and after treatment.

HYPOTHERMIA

This can be a sign of cold environment or of serious systemic infection. Severe hypothermia happens when temperature is less than 90⁰F. Between 90⁰F to 96⁰F, hypothermia is moderate.

Severe hypothermia may need air heated incubator. Otherwise following steps should be taken.

- Child's cold clothing should be removed and replaced with prewarmed clothes.
- Hot water bottle may be used under the blanket.
- For skin to skin rewarming, place the infant between the mother's breasts.
- Continue feeding to prevent drop in blood glucose level.

POLIOMYELITIS

This is an acute viral disease affecting the spinal cord and motor nerve cells in the brain stem. There are three known strains of virus I, II and III. The virus enters the body orally along with contaminated food and water.

What are its clinical features?

Initial symptoms are like that of flu, sudden fever, headache, sore throat, vomiting etc. lasting for a day. Then the child will have high fever, vomiting, stiffness of neck, muscular pain and rigidity for a few days. In the next few days a paralytic phenomenon sets in. Most often the leg muscles are affected.

(i) In the spinal type, paralysis involves groups of limb muscles and is typically symmetrical. Leg muscles become flaccid with loss of tendon reflexes and subsequent wasting. Sensations are not affected.

(ii) In bulbar type there may be weakness of the facial muscle's, difficulty in swallowing, nasal voice, difficulty in chewing, dribbling of saliva and nasal regularitation. There may be paralysis even of the respiratory system. Here tracheostomy has to be done.

How to manage a case of poliomyelitis?

- Complete bed rest for 2-3 weeks so long there is no fever and pain.
- The child's position should be neutral to prevent deformities. Affected side should be supported by pillows.
- Foot drop should be prevented with help of a padded splint.
- Hospitalisation may be required.

How to relieve pain?

- Suitable analgesics, i.e. paracetamol, ibuprofen, may be given in suitable doses.

- Diazepam pediatric syrup may be given.
- Nutrition should be adequately maintained.

How physiotherapy helps?

Daily gentle massage and passive movements are to be practiced from the begining. After apparent recovery there should be graded physiotherapy directly under an expert physiotherapist.

CONSTIPATION

It refers to the passage of small, hard, dry stools that contain much of solids and minimal water.

What are the fundamental factors contributing to constipation?

There are two factors –

- Defects in emptying the rectum.
- Defects in filling the rectum. Both in defective emptying and filling excessive drying of stool follows. Hard, dry stools are rather painful to evacuate leading to further retention. Constipation therefore tends to be self-perpetuating.

What type of constipation develops in neonatal and early infancy?

In infancy breast fed babies may pass stools only once in a few days. This stool in generally loose and seldom dry. If a breast fed infant's mother is consuming enough fats and proteins his stools may be firmer and pultaceous.

Artificial feeding, inadequate fluid intake, especially in hot whether or excessive sweating due to over clothing, or inadequate sugar in milk feed may all lead to constipation.

Certain drugs and excessive abuse of laxatives may lead to constipation.

What are the causes of constipation in later infancy and childhood?

Inadequate dietary roughage and large amounts of milk are by far the most common cause.

Parents eager to have their child have a bowel movement daily, indulge in frequent administration of laxatives to the child. As a result he becomes dependent on drugs.

Inadequate dietary roughage and large amounts of milk are the most common cause of constipation.

How can poor toilet training affect?

Overanxious parents may force the child to sit on the pottie far too long against the child's wish. Others may examine each and every stool critically, inducing the child to refuse to empty his bowels.

Reactive constipation secondary to poor toilet is most often seen in children whose mothers are overprotective, tense and anxious and who's fathers, on the other hand, are fond of exerting excessive discipline.

CONVULSIONS

Convulsions are a temporary disturbance of brain function manifested by involuntary motor, sensory, autonomic or psychic phenomenon. These becomes irritation of CNS.

When are convulsions likely to develop?

The peak incidence occurs during the first 2 years. Disorders stimulating recurrent convulsions include breath holding spells, hysterical fits, migraine, syncope and apneic spells.

What are the types of convulsions that may develop?

In the newborn it is frequent to see convulsions in the form of typical tonic and clonic movements. Some may have twitchings, conjugate deviations of eyes, irregular jerky movements and nystagmus. Feeble cry and cyanotic attacks may well mean convulsions.

What types of convulsions take place in new born?

- First and second day – Birth injury, axphyxia, hypoxia, intracranial hemorrhage vitamin B_6 deficiency, inborn errors of metabolism all may lead it.
- Third day – Hypoglycemia may cause it.
- Fourth day and onwards – Septicemia, meningitis, hypocalcemic tetany may cause it.

What perinatal problems may cause it?

Birth trauma following difficult delivery are a common cause. Convulsions may present as tonic spasms, preceded by some clonic jerks on the first day only.

Can hypocalcaemia cause convulsions?

It occurs usually in babies on cow's milk formula rich in phosphates. Manifestations occur on I^{st} day or 7th day of birth. Serum calcium is below 8 mg%.

Intravenous injection of 5 to 10 ml 10% solution of calcium gluconate leads to dramatic response.

Can hypoglycemia result in convulsions?

It develops in infants who suffer from intrauterine growth retardation. In infants of diabetic or prediabetic mothers, in smaller or twins and in respiratory distress syndrome it can develop. Blood level goes below 30 mg % and manifestations include tremors, cyanosis and apneic spells.

What infections may result in convulsions?

- Tetanus is likely to occur in new born in whom the umbilical cord is cut under septic conditions, or be infected by mud and dung. It usually manifests 5 or 6 days after birth with difficulty in sucking, stiffness of jaws and generalised spasticity.

CONVULSIONS IN CHILDHOOD

The term refers to seizures occuring at the onset of extra eranial infection or in association with hot wheather.

What are febrile convulsions?

Salient features of it are –

- Generalised rather than focal convulsions.
- Attack lasts less than 10 minutes and in no case more than 20 minutes.
- There is no recurrence before 12-18 hours of attack.
- There is no paralysis.
- It is accompanied with rapid rise of temperature.
- CSF and EEC are normal.

Can pyogenic meningitis result in convulsions?

It may manifest suddenly with convulsions in association with high fever, irritability, vomiting, headache and neck stiffness. Presence of generalised purpuric rash points to meningococcal meningitis.

Can convulsions develop in encephalitis?

Encephalitis manifests with change in sensorium, fever, vomiting, in addition to convulsions. Infants may show gross irritability. There may be peculiar behaviour and altered speech.

What type of convulsions results in cerebral abscess?

It is characterized by headache, vomiting and visual disturbance. High or low irregular fever, chills, rigors, irritability and behavioral problems may develop from it.

Can certain drugs lead to convulsions?

The list of drugs include phenothiazines, antihistamines, steroids, acetazolamide, chloroquine, nalidixic acid, etc.

EPILEPSY

(i) Grand Mal – Convulsions are predominantly tonic during infancy. There is an 'aura'. Aura includes warning signals of epilepsy. During the tonic phase of less than 20-40 seconds child loses consciousness. His face becomes pale, distorted and eyeballs rolls up. The pupils dilate and cornea becomes insensitive to touch. Rapid contractions of jaw muscles may cause biting of tongue.

After the attack the patient generally falls asleep.

(ii) Petitmal epilepsy – Dizzy spells, fainting, transient lapses of consciousness for a few seconds without an aura, i.e. previous warning takes place. He may drop the pen/note book held in his hand during the attack. The child is unaware of the attacks. Disco lights and sounds may precipitate it.

It does not occur before the age of 3 years and often settles by puberty. Peak incidence takes place between 4 and 8 years.

(iii) Focal epilepsy – It may be motor or sensory. In motor, variety convulsions are clonic. Hand, face and tongue are affected usually. Convulsions beginning in thumb spread to fingers, wrist and arm.

(iv) Psychomotor epilepsy – This is characterized by nausea, vomiting or epigastric sensation followed by a short period of increased muscular tonicity. Some children may have slight aura. Episode remains for 1-5 minutes.

(v) Infantile myoclonic epilepsy – Massive attack of sudden dropping of head and flexion of arm before the age of 2 years. There may be associated mental retardation.

FAILURE TO THRIVE

It refers to infants and children who fail to gain weight proportional to height and age.

Can nutritional deprivation lead to it?

Gross deficiency of protein and energy intake may cause retarded growth. Nutritional dwarfing is a common problem in our conditions. Affected child is less lively and less active and is more prone to diarrhoea, pneumonia or tuberculosis.

Can maternal/social/environmental deprivation lead to it?

Emotional deprivation resulting from psychosocial circumstances may affect the child's intake.

How do intestinal parasites affect the growth of a child?

It is one of the leading cause.

(i) Chronic giardiasis – This is characterized by vague upper abdominal pain and recurrent diarrhoea.

(ii) Ascariasis – There will be growth failure, abdominal distension, pain, anemia, vitamin deficiency and voracious appetite. Some may develop sleeplessness, irritability, urticaria, and eosinophilia. Occasionally intestinal obstruction may develop. Liver and spleen may enlarge.

(iii) Hook worm infestation – There will be progressive anemia, loss of appetite, pain in the abdomen and malnutrition. The child may eat unusual things like mud, chalk, etc. Child may develop generalised oedema. Diarrhoea with alternative constipation may be present.

How will tuberculosis affect?

Undiagnosed primary complex may be responsible for a good proportion to cause failure to thrive. In addition there will be malaise, fatigue, weight loss and low grade fever. X-ray of chest may show the lesion.

DYSPNEA

There is a difficulty in breathing. It may develop at rest or on exertion.

What is the respiratory distress syndrome?

This may occur in a preterm baby. It usually occurs in first hour of birth with increasing, respiratory distress. Grunting respiration, flaring of nostrils, retraction of ribs and cyanosis are usually present. Low blood pressure, hypothermia and hemorrhagic manifestation may complicate the picture.

Can massive aspiration of fluid result in dyspnea?

There may be massive amount of amniotic fluid, blood or meconium aspirated in breech presentation, forceps delivery or prolonged labour. At birth the baby will be asphyxiated and shocked. There will be a high pitched cry.

During feeds the baby gets chocked or regurgitates.

What is an intrauterine pneumonia?

Intrauterine pneumonia may occur in prolonged delivery, premature rupture of membranes and birth asphyxia.

The baby is ill, depressed and lethargic at birth. He is not interested in sucking the breast. About 12-18 hours after birth he becomes dysponeic. Respiration is often grunting.

Can pneumothorax develop dysponeia?

Pneumothorax occurs in newborns more often than at any other stage. Fetal distress or a difficult delivery leading to aspiration of meconium results in this. Along with this dyspnea cyanosis develops. X-ray confirms diagnosis.

Can tracheosophageal fistula result it?

Newborn develops excessive drooling called, 'blowing bubbles', coughing, gagging and even chocking. Milk and saliva may regurgitate and enter the lungs causing aspiration pneumonia.

POSTENEONATAL PERIOD

How does bronchial asthma affect?

Temporary narrowing of bronchi by bronchospasm, mucosal oedema and thick secretions lead to bouts of dysponea. Onset of paroxysm is usually sudden, often ocuring at night. The child may develop tightness in chest.

A typical attack consists of marked dysponea, bouts of cough and wheezing. Cyanosis, pallor, sweating, exhaustion and restlessness are present. Pulse becomes rapid. Attack may subside in an hour or so.

What is bronchiolitis?

It is a serious disease of bronchioles of viral origin specially at the age of 6 months. The child develops catarrh, dysponea and postration. Breathing is rapid and shallow. Mild to moderate fever is present. Cough when present is minimal.

This needs a medical care.

How pneumonia develops into fever?

Dysponea is of acute onset. It is accompanied with high fever, chills and cough. There will be grunting expiration. X-ray gives diagnosis.

What is an asthmatic bronchitis?

Dysponea is a feature of asthmatic bronchitis. It develops in the first 2 years of life. The child develops significant bronchospasm.

Can a child develop tropical eosinophilia?

This disease, beyond 1 year of age, develops with some exertional dysponea, persistent cough, wheeze, low fever, growth retardation and weakness. There may be enlargement of liver and glands.

Why pleural effucion results in dysponeia?

After the age of 5 years it develops from discharge of caseous material. There may be fever, weight loss and chest pain.

Can there be a congenital lobar emphysema?

The child may present with dysponea and cyanosis following compression of normal lung by emphysematous lung.

TUBERCULOSIS

What is Ghon's focus?

When a person is infected by tubercle bacilli for the first time, there develops a minute primary tubercular lesion at the site of the lodgement of bacilli. Incubation period is 12 weeks. Ghon's focus appears as a subpleural lesion more commonly in apical region of lung.

Ordinarily this may heal automatically due to natural immunity. If not healed this may cause cough and cold, fever and failure to thrive. If not treated this may lead to tubercular meningitis.

How to confirm the diagnosis of T.B.?

Followings test will be helpful

(i) Strongly positive tuberculin test – Mantoux test with 10 m.m. or more induration is the most important diagnostic criterion test.

(ii) In doubtful cases Elisa test of blood for detection of antitubercular antibody can be resorted to.

(iii) E.S.R. more than 20 m.m. per hour.

(iv) X-ray chest.

How to manage a case of T.B.?

- Bed rest and a high protein diet.
- Rifampicin, isoniazid and pyrizinamide combinations are suitable for 3 months.
- Later on Rifampicin and isoniazid can be continued for another 3 to 6 months.

BURNS AND SCALDS

What do you understand by burns?

Burns are the injuries that result from dry heat like fire, flame, piece of hot metal, sun, lightening and friction.

Scalds are the injuries caused by moist heat like boiling water, steam, oil, hot tar and hot liquids.

What are the dangers of burns?

- Infection – There is a big risk of infection with burns because skin is damaged and there is no protection against the germs.
- Shock – Shock develops because blood serum leaks out of circulatory system into the burnt area.

How is burn graded?

- Area wise – Burns are classified on the basis of area by rule of 9. Any burn of over 30% needs hospitalization.

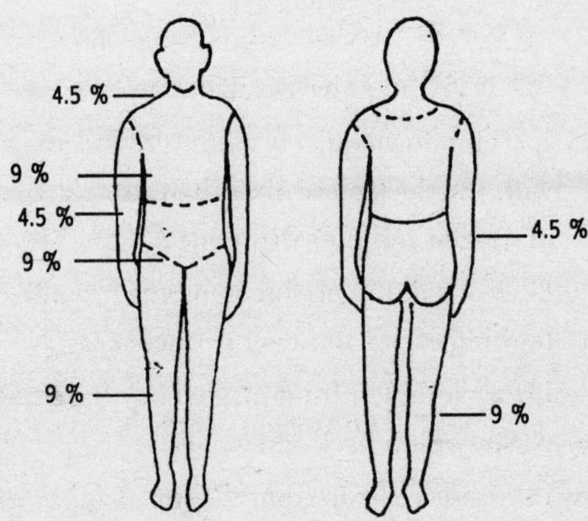

AREAS DIVIDED FOR CALCULATION OF BURNS

- Burns larger than 2.5 cm square requires medical attention.

What are signs and symptoms of burns?

- There will be severe pain in and around the injured area if it is a superficial burn.
- Redness and swelling of area.
- Blisters are thin bubbles which form on the skin damaged by heat. These are caused by tissue fluid leaking into the burnt area just under the surface of skin.
- Grey charred skin around deep burn.
- Blood pressure and pulse falls.

How to help a person who has caught fire?

- Most of the burn occurs at home and drinking water is readily available to quench the flames. Water also cools the area.
- Do not allow the person to run around. This only fans the fire and makes the flames spread.
- Hold a rug, blanket, coat in front while approaching person whose clothings have caught fire.
- Lay him down quickly on the ground and wrap him tightly with any thick piece of cloth or coat. This starves the flames of oxygen and puts them out.
- Do not roll the person along the ground as this can cause burning of previously unharmed areas.
- If the clothes in front of the body have caught fire, lay the person on his back and vice versa.

How to rescue a person from the site of a fire?

- Clean air is at ground level. So crawl along the floor to pull out a person who is lying disabled.
- Have a wet handkerchief round your face when you rescue.
- Quick action is needed because room may have some amount of carbon mono oxide gas.

What is the treatment of minor burns?

- Reassure the casuality. Place the injured part under slowly running cold water or immerse it in cold water for ten minutes.
- Gently remove ring, watch, shoes and other constricting clothes from the injured area before it starts to swell.
- Dress the area with clean, sterile material.

- Do not use adhensive dressing.
- Do not allow cotton wool.
- Do not break blisters.

ELECTRICAL INJURIES

Electrical shock is produced when an electric current passes through the human body which is in contact with earth. It passes even more quickly if the part is wet.

In wet conditions even lower voltage may be dangerous. A very strong current passing to earth through lower limbs may be less dangerous than a weaker current passing through the chest specially when it enters through the hands and arms.

What are the signs and symptoms of electric shock?

- There may be sudden stoppage of breathing due to paralysis of muscles used in breathing.
- The heart may continue to beat but breathing has stopped. There may be blueness of face.
- There may be superficial or deep burns.
- Fatal paralysis of heart.

How you will manage a case of electric injury?

Intelligent and prompt action is required. If the first aider is not cautious he may also receive severe electric shock or even die along with the casualty.

- Switch off the current if the casuality is still in contact with the conductor. If switch is not to be found, remove the plug or cut off the current by breaking the wire. You have to stand on a dry piece of wooden board. Do not use scissors or knife. First aider should keep as far away as possible from electric wires because current can pass through the gap resulting in an arc.

- If casuality is not breathing normally or heart has stopped give artificial respiration and external cardiac massage.
- Treat for shock.
- Treat for burns if any.

What about electrical burns?

- Burns may occur when high voltage current passes through the body.
- Much damage occurs at point of entry but at exit only small burns may be visible but damage to the underlying tissues may be considerable.
- Redness, swelling, charring of skin at both the entry and exit points.
- Breathing and heart may have stopped.
- Symptoms of shock are noted.

Separate the casuality from the source of injury. Place a sterile dressing over the injury and shift the patient to hospital. Do not break blisters. Do not remove any loose skin.

FOREIGN BODIES

1. Swallowed Foreign Bodies

- Smooth, small foreign bodies do not cause much alarm. (small coin, small button)
- Sharp object on the other hand cause severe damage as pins or needles.

- Always shift to medical care.
- Do not give anything by mouth.

2. **Foreign bodies in nose**

- Small object may lodge itself in the nose but sharp objects may damage the nostrils.
- There will be difficulty in breathing.
- Nose appears swollen

Such patient should be taken to the hospital.

3. **Foreign bodies in ear**

- Insects may get lodged in ear
- There will be pain in ear.
- Vibrations if insects are inside ear.
- Gently flood the ear with water. Do not use force.
- Consult a doctor.

4. **Foreign bodies in eyes**

- All eye injuries are serious because particles may perforate the eye ball and cause infection.
- Particles of dust or loose eye lashes are commonly found in eyes sticking at the outer surface of eye ball.
- There will be pain and itching in the eyes.
- Vision may be impaired. Redness of eye develops.

How will you manage?

- Do not to rub eyes.
- If foreign body is visible, wash the eye with sterile water. Incline the head towards the injured eye.
- If foreign body cannot be removed, cover the affected eye with an eye pad. Secure it lightly and consult the doctor.

EFFECT OF TEMPERATURE

SUN BURN

Direct exposure to sun rays may cause sun burn. Windy climate and winter on high mountains predisposes it

What will be the signs of sun burn?

- Skin is red, swollen and painful.
- Itching over the burn.
- Affected skin will become hot.

How will you manage?

- Remove the patient to a cool place.
- Sponging with cold water.
- Cream in any form can be applied.
- Give sips of cold water frequently.

HYPOTHERMIA

This condition develops when body temperature falls below 95^0C. Moderate hypothermia can be reversed. But below 85^0F is unlikely to improve.

How does hypothermia develop?

It can develop in the following cases –

- Environment temperature is low.
- Prolonged immersion in cold water.
- Exhaustation in cold climate.
- Wearing wet clothes for long.
- High cold altitude.

Condition is aggrevated by consumption of alcohol and diabetes in old age.

What are its symptoms?

- Feeling very cold.
- Skin becomes very pale.
- Intense shivering.
- Muscle incoordination and slurred speech.
- Restlessness, irritability and confusion.
- Loss of consciousness.
- Breathing becomes difficult.

How will you manage a case of hypothermia?

- Never assume that the body is dead even if respiration and heart beat is not felt.
- Cover the casuality with woolen cloth except the face.
- Unconscious casuality should be placed in recovery position.
- Keep a person in a warm room.
- Give sweet drinks.
- Shift to hospital.

FORST BITE

Frost bite occurs when ears, nose, chin, hands and feet are exposed to intense cold for long.

There are two types of frost bite

(i) Superficial skin freeze.

(ii) Deep skin and underlying tissues being frozen.

What are its sign and symptoms?

There will be

- Prickling pain in the affected part.
- Gradual development of numbness.
- Impairement and stiffness of part involved.
- Skin changes in mottled blue colour.

How will you treat such patients?

- Remove the casuality to a shelter.
- Remove constrictive things.
- Warm the part with your warm skin.
- Elevate the affected part with pillow etc. to relieve pain and swelling.
- Shift the patient to hospital.

HEAT EXHAUSTION

It occurs after heavy and prolonged sweating with failure to replace salt and water in hot climate. It generally occurs in hot and humid climate.

What are its clinical features?

- Exhaustion and restlessness.
- Frontal headache.
- Tiredness, nausea, dizziness.
- Skin becomes cold and pale.
- Person feels muscle cramps in lower limbs.
- Temperature may be normal/subnormal.
- Pulse is rapid and weak.
- Fast and shallow breathing.

How you will manage such cases?

- Remove patient to a cooler place in fresh air.
- Lay him down and loosen all clothing.
- Give cold water to drink with little salt and sugar.
- Give crocin tablet and do sponging.

HEAT STROKE

This occurs when body can no longer control its temperature by sweating. It may be caused by exposure to heat and humidity.

What are its clinical features?

- Headache, dizziness.
- Restlessness, nausea and vomiting.
- Skin remains dry. Body temperature is above 105^{0}F.
- No sweating.
- Muscular cramps.
- Full and bounding pulse.
- Noisy breathing.

How will you manage it?

- Wrap the casuality in a cold wet sheet and keep him wet.
- Fan should be on.
- Cold sponging should be started.
- Replace the body fluids.
- Apply ice cap.
- When temperature comes down to 102^{0}F and person is concious stop sponging.

MALNUTRITION

Malnutrition can be due to improper or inadequate food intake. It may also result from inadequate absorption of food. Deficient supply of food, poor dietary habits, food faddism and emotional factors may also limit food intake.

How you will classify malnutrition?

Marasmus – Lack of calories.

Kwashiorkor – Mainly lack of proteins and calories.

Obesity – Excessive consumption of calories than required.

MARASMUS

What is marasmus?

Clinical reason of marasmus is due to general starvation. It may be due to inadequate intake of calories or due to improper feeding habits.

What are the clinical features of marasmus?

There is failure to gain weight followed by loss of weight until obivious emaciation results. Skin becomes wrinkled due to loose subcutaneous fat. Fat becomes shrunken and child looks intelligent and loooks like a monkey face. Abdomen may be distended. Appetite may be increased or decreased or reduced with occasional diarrhoea. There may be associated vitamin deficiency.

KWASHIORKOR

The child becomes apathetic, anaemic, anorexic and oedematous. He develops diarrhoea. There is growth retardation. Child looses

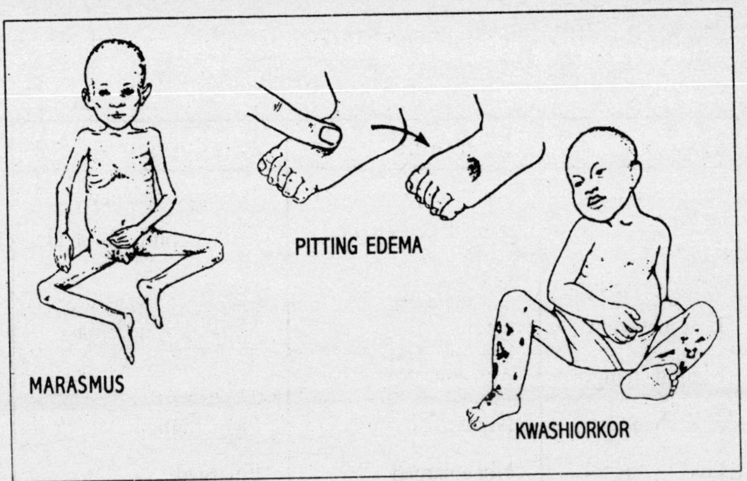

weight but due to oedema he does not look skinny. There may be ascites.

What type of skin changes takes place?

Skin changes may involve any part of body specially lower limbs. Darkening of skin appears in areas of irritation but not in those exposed to sunlight. There may be areas of pigmentation and depigmentation. Cracks appear at folds and ulcer may develop. Hair becomes brown and coarse.

What is the difference between Marasmus and Kwashiorkor?

Difference between Marasmus/kwashiorkor

Feature	Marasmus	Kwashiorkor
Cause wasting	Deficiency of calories	Protein deficiency
	Thin, lean and skiny	Flabby child, Moon face
Muscle wasting	Severe	Less
Loss of weight	Severe	Marked by oedema
Mental changes	Abscent	Present
Skin changes	None	Pigmentation
Liver	Not enlarged	Enlarged
Hair changes	Slight change	Brownish, sparsh

What is the cheapest treatment?

National institute of nutrition has developed the following mixture

Whole wheat roasted	40 gram
Ground nut roasted	10 gram
Bengal gram roasted	16 gram
Jaggery	20 gram

Total weight	86 gram
Energy	330 Kcal
Protein	11.3 gram

This mixture should be given for three months.

OBESITY

Obesity is the bank balance of calories. A child who is obese will only become an obese adult. Obesity leads to many diseases such as diabetes, heart problem, the kidney ailments and arthritis etc. From the very begining the weight of the child should be controlled keeping a check on ice creams and fatty fried foods.

Standard Height and Weights for Adult Indian Men and Women

Height (feet)	Men (Weight in Kilogram)	Women (Weight in Kilogram)
(5'-0")	–	50.8—54.4
(5'-1")	–	51.7—55.3
(5'-2")	56.3—60.3	53.1—56.7
(5'-3")	57.6—61.7	54.4—58.9
(5'-4")	58.9—63.5	56.3—59.9
(5'-5")	60.8—65.3	57.6—61.2
(5'-6")	62.2—66.7	58.9—63.5
(5'-8")	64.0—68.5	60.8—65.3
(5'-9")	65.8—70.8	62.2—66.7
(5'-10")	67.6-—72.6	64.0—68.5
(5'-11")	69.4—74.4	65.8—70.3
(6'-0")	71.2—76.2	67.1—71.7
(6'-1")	73.0—78.5	68.5—73.9
(6'-2")	75.3—80.7	

(Compiled from the Standard set by the Life Insurance Corporation of India)

Average Height and Weight for Indian Children

Age Group	Boys			Girls		
	Height		Weight	Height		Weight
	cms	ft. in	kgs.	cms	ft.in	kgs
Up to 3 months	56.2	1-10	4.5	55.0	1-10	4.2
4-6 months	62.7	2-1	6.7	60.9	2-0	5.6
7-9 months	64.9	2-2	6.9	64.4	2-2	6.2
10-12 months	69.5	2-4	7.4	66.7	2-2½	6.6
1 year	73.9	2-5½	8.4	72.5	2-5	7.8
2 years	81.6	2-8½	10.1	80.1	2-8	9.6
3 years	88.8	2-11½	11.8	87.2	2-11	11.2
4 years	96.0	3-2	13.5	94.5	3-2	12.9
5 years	102.1	3-5	14.8	101.4	3-4½	14.5
6 years	108.5	3-7	16.3	107.4	3-7	16.0
7 years	113.9	3.9½	18.0	112.8	3.9	17.6
8 years	119.3	4-0	19.7	118.2	3-11	19.4
9 years	123.7	4-1½	21.5	122.9	4-1	21.3
10 years	128.4	4-3	23.5	128.4	4-3	23.6
11 years	133.4	4-5	25.9	133.6	4-5½	26.4
12 years	138.3	4-7½	28.5	139.2	4-7½	29.8
13 years	144.6	4-10	32.1	143.9	4-9½	33.3
14 years	150.1	5-0	35.7	147.5	4.11	36.8
15 years	155.5	5-2	39.6	149.6	5-0	36.8
16 years	159.5	5-4	43.2	151.0	5-½	41.1
17 years	161.4	5-5½	45.7	151.5	5-½	42.4

(Compiled by the Statistics Division of The Indian Council of Medical Research, New Delhi).

TONSILLITIS

Tonsils are made of lymphatic material and form a part of body's natural defence mechanism. These are bodyguards of the body and fight unwelcome germs entering the body. These start smaller after the age of 7 years.

What is acute tonsillitis?

This is very common in children below 10 years. It spreads by droplets. It may be caused by bacteria or virus.

What are its signs and symptoms?

The child goes off his food and finds swallowing painful. There may be headache or earache. The child appears hot and flushed. Lymph glands of neck may be enlarged. Tonsils become large, red, strawberry like with streaks or white spots.

How to manage tonsillitis?

Suitable antibiotics will help. Control fever with paracetamol. Give lots of fluids. Do not give icecreams.

When should tonsils be removed?

Tonsils are a useful and protective part of the young body and are worth keeping. If tonsils are removed children get frequent infection of throat.

But if a child gets more than 4 attacks of tonsillitis in a year for 3 years, removal of tonsils may prove useful.

SPRAIN

This is the result of tearing or stretching of a ligament of a joint. The fibrous capsule that encloses the joint is damaged. Ankle is mostly affected.

Movement increases the pain. X-ray is done to rule out fracture. Treatment with ice packs for 48 hours and drugs like brufamol will help.

FRACTURE

Fracture is the partial or complete breakage of periosteum. Any direct or indirect force can lead to a fracture.

What are the types of fracture?

- Simple (closed fracture). In this fracture the skin surface around the damaged bone is not broken.
- Compound (open fracture). When the wound leads from the surface.
- Complicated fracture – closed or open fractures are said to be complicated when there is an associated injury, i.e. an injury to a vessel and nerves.

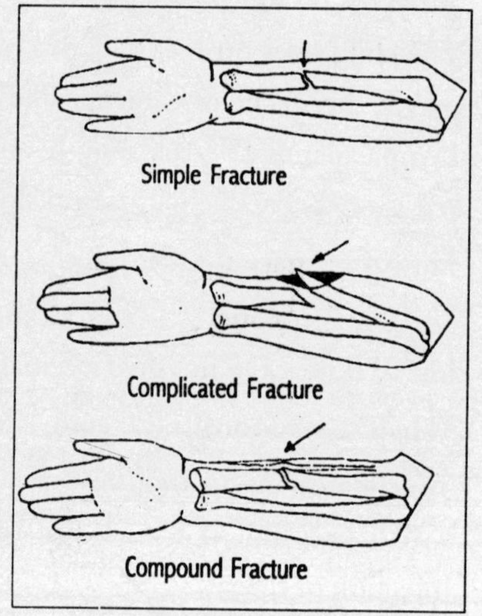

What are the signs and symptoms of fracture?

- Pain at or near the site of injury, which increases with movement.
- Difficulty in movement.

- Swelling of the area and discolouration.
- Deformity.
- Tenderness.
- Signs of shock if too much bleeding has taken place.

How to manage a case of fracture?

- Immobilize and support the fractured limb using bandages or splints. This should be done on both sides of fracture, above and below it.

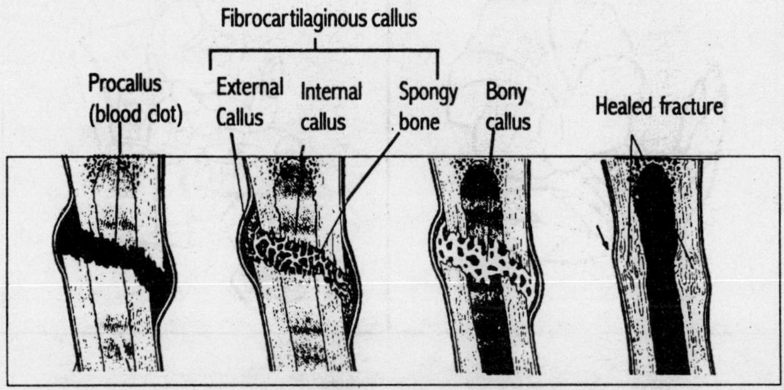

DIFFERENT STAGES OF HEALING OF FRACTIONS

- Do not apply tight bandage directly over the area of fracture.
- At other places the bandage should be fairly firm so that there is no movement of the fractured ends.
- Splint is a rigid piece of wood or plastic material or metal applied to a fractured limb. Resonably wide splints give better support.
- Raise the injured part after splinting.
- Consult a doctor.

How much time does it takes for a fracture to heal?

It takes about 14 days to start callus at the point of fracture and another 2 to 4 weeks to heal the fracture. Some calcium preparation should be taken at thus time.

What are minor cuts?

Minor cuts are where the skin is cut but no big blood vessel is torn or ruptured. After cleaning the wound a band-aid may be applied. Such injuries do not require stitches.

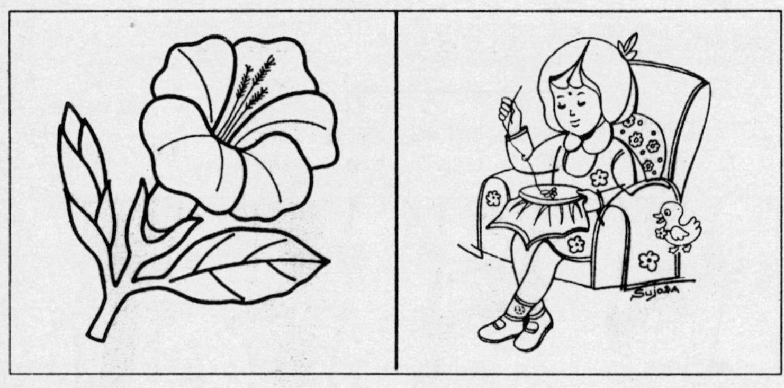

Common Drugs and Doses

Dr. Rahul Jain

Warning – Doctor should be consulted before these drugs are given in the greater interest of child.

To control fever

- Paracetamol. (Crocin, Calpol, Metacin Pyrigesic.)

It is used to bring down high fever. Dose is 40-60 mg/kg/day, 4-6 hourly.

To control intestinal worms

- Albendazole (Zentel, Wormin, Albendazole)

This is used for pinworm, roundworm, hookworm.

Dose 200 mg single dose between 1-2 years, 400 mg single dose for children above 2 years. Repeat dose after 2 weeks.

- Piperazine salts (Antepar, piperazine citrate syrup).

This is used in ascariasis.

Dose 75 mg/kg/day orally as single dose.

Antibiotics

- Cephalexin (Cephaxin, Sepaxin. Sporidex syrup 125 mg per ml, drops 100 mg per ml.)

Dose 25-50 mg/kg/day 6 hourly.

- Ciprofloxacin (Cifran, Ciproflox)

This should be given when other antibiotics have failed.

Dose 20-30 mg/kg/day 12 hourly, orally.

- Norfloxacin (Norflox, Norbid)

In urinary tract infection.

Dose 10-15 mg/kg/day 12 hourly.

- Erythromycin (Althrocin, E-mycin, Erythrocin)

Dose 30-50 mg/kg/day 6 hourly, orally.

- Amoxycillin (Novamox, Amoxyban)

Dose 25-30 mg/kg/day 8 hourly, orally.

Anti emetic

- Domperidone (Domstal, Emitin,)

It is used in vomiting.

Dose 0.2-0.4 mg/kg/ every 4-8 hour.

- Metoclopramide hydrochloride (Perinorm, Maxeron, Reglan)

This is used to check vomiting.

Dose 0.1 mg/kg/ 6-8 hourly, orally.

Antiallergic

- Chlorpheniramine maleate – (Piriton Polaramine)

Dose 2-6 years – 1 mg; 6-12 years 2 mg

- Promethazine hydrochloride (Phenargan, elixir 5 mg per ml)

For nausea and vomiting – 0.25-1 mg/k/g 4-6 hourly, orally.

For motion sickness 0.5 mg/kg/ dose 12 hourly, orally.

Antimalarial

- Chloroquin phosphate (Cloquin, Nivaquin, Emquin)

Dose – 10 mg of base/kg oral stat. Followed by 5 mg/kg at 6

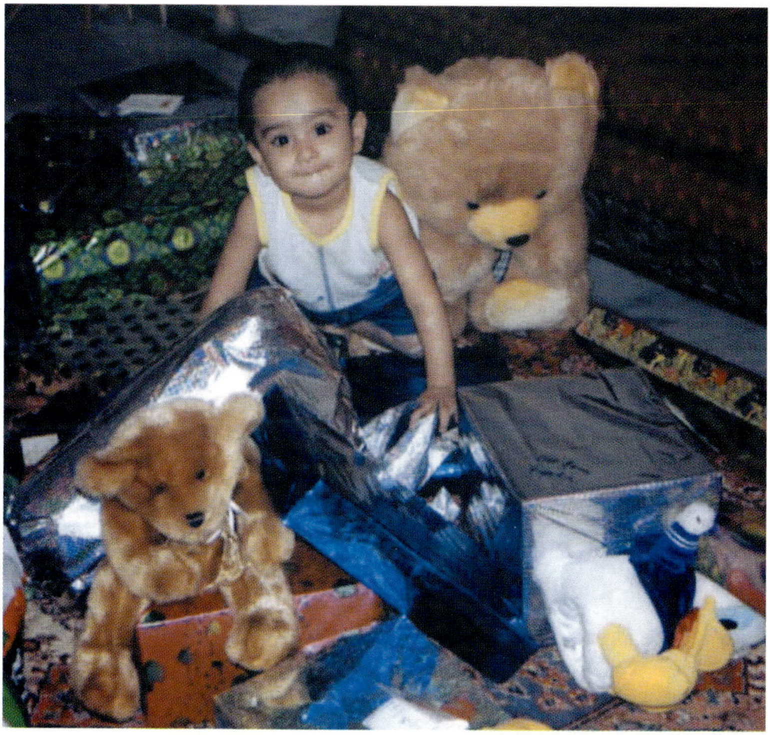

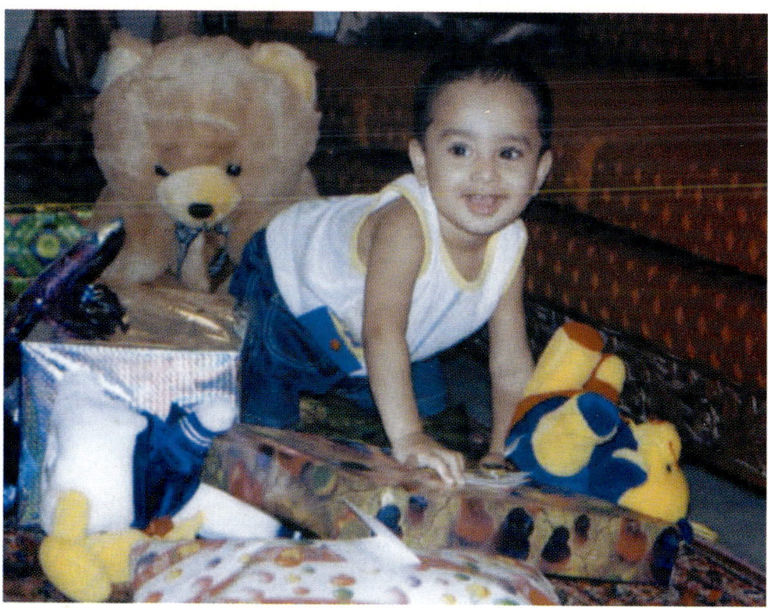

Playing with toys.

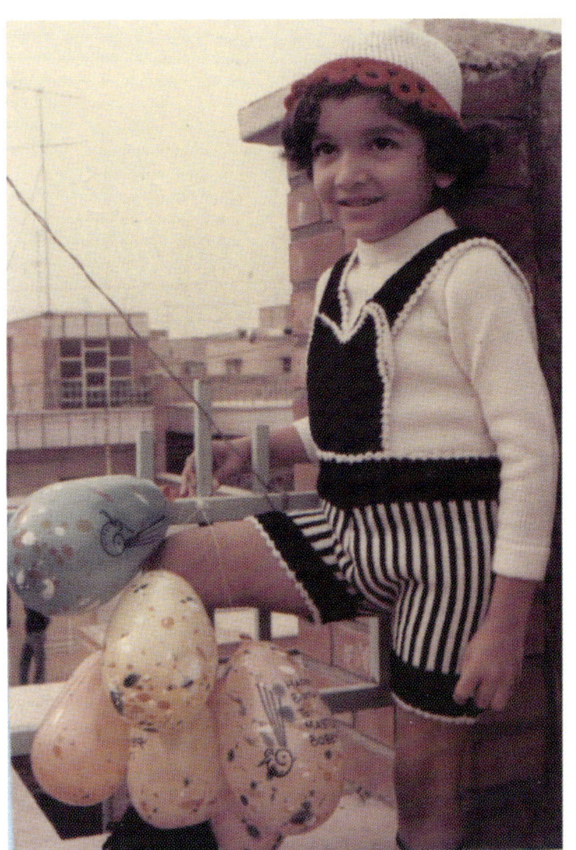

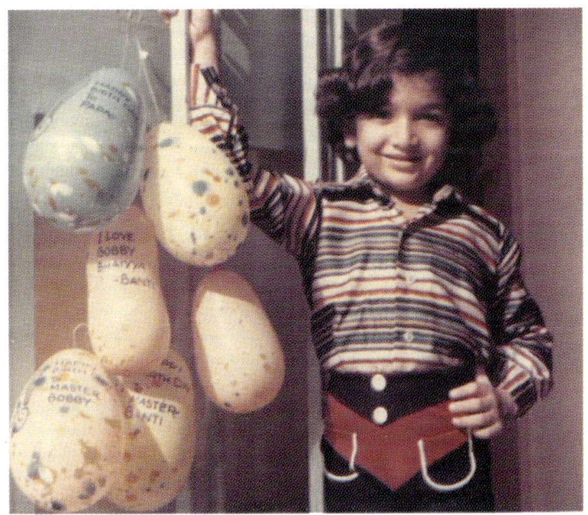

Coloured baloons are their valuables

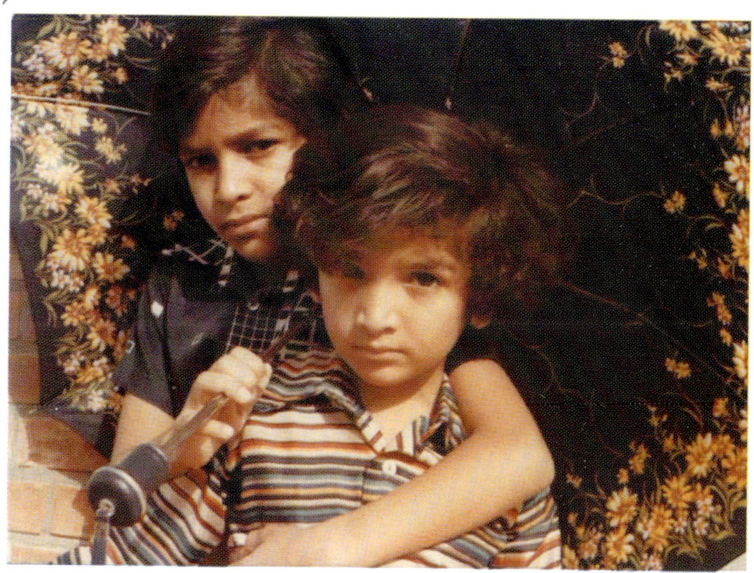

Child's rivalry ends at 'five'.

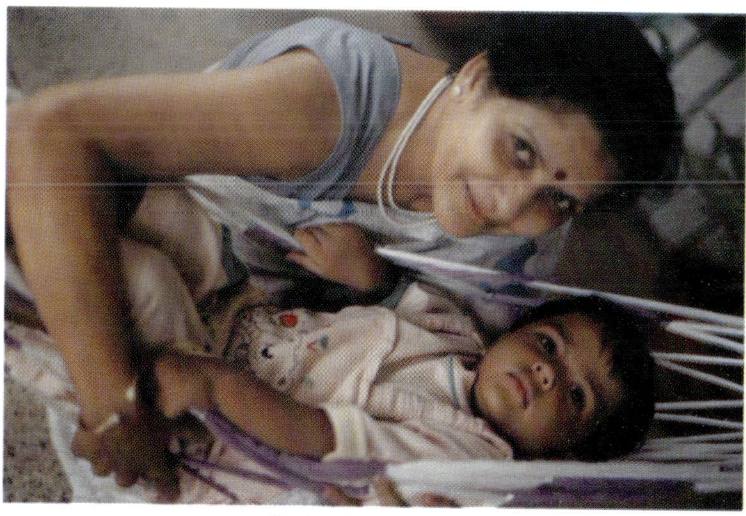

Swinging is a joy.

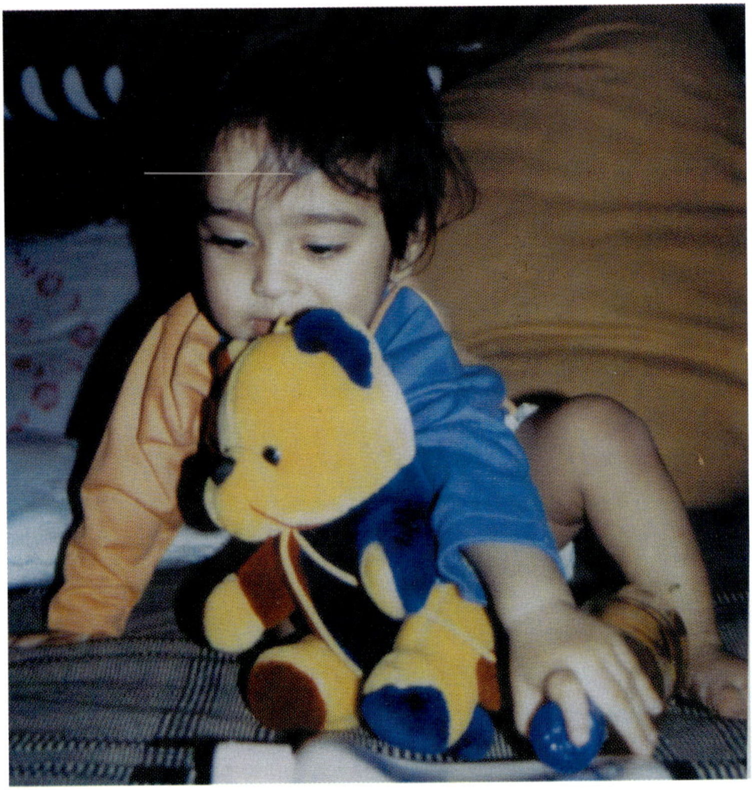

Busy with toy.

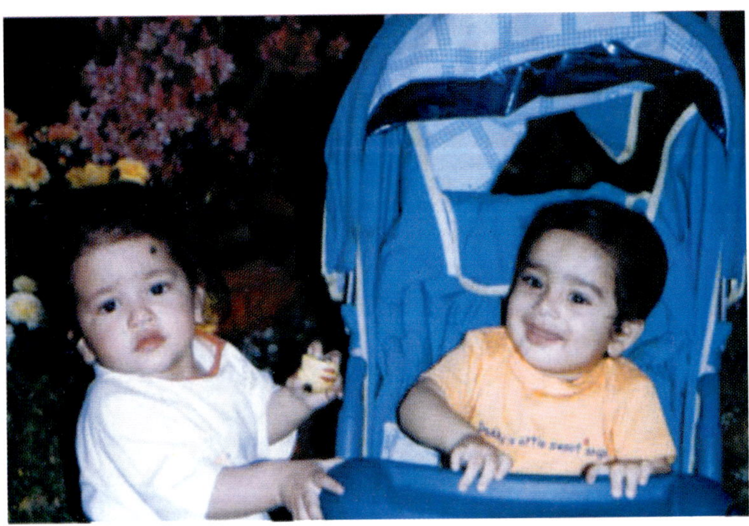

Child is fond of company of his own.

hour, 24 hour and 48 hour. Total dose 25 mg/kg within 48 hours. Fox prophylaxis of malaria 5 mg/kg once a week.

- Melfloquine hydrochloride – (Mefloc, Mefque, Larimex)

It is used in drug resistant uncomplicated P. falciparum malaria 1.5 mg/kg single dose orally. Second dose of 10 mg/kg is given 8-24 hours later.

- Pyrimethamine (Metakelfin, Malarwin)

For treatment of chloroquin resistant uncomplicated P. falciparum. Dose – 1 mg/kg as single dose.

Antiprotozoal agents

- Metronidazole (Flagyl, aristogyl).

Dose 15-20 mg/kg/day 8 hourly, orally for 10 days for giardiasis.

Dose 35-50 mg/kg/day 8 hourly, orally for 10 days in amoebiasis.

Antitubercular agents

- Isoniazid – 5-10 mg/kg//day. Single dose daily. (Isonex forte tab 300 mg).
- Pyrazinamide (Pyzin, PZA-ciba 250 mg/5ml).

Dose 20-35 mg/kg/day single dose daily.

- Rifampicin (R-cinex kid tab, Tricinex kid tab).

Dose 10 mg/kg/day single dose on empty stomach.

Antispasmodics (to control pain in the abdomen)

- Dicyclomine Hydrochloride – (Colimex, Spasmindon.

Dose – infants below 6 months 5-10 drops, 15 minutes before feed.

6 months-2 years 10 to 20 drops.

- Oxyphenonium bromide (Antrenyl drops 20 mg/ml, 5 and 10 mg tablet.

Dose – 0.8 mg/kg/day 6 hourly 5-10 drops in preschool children.

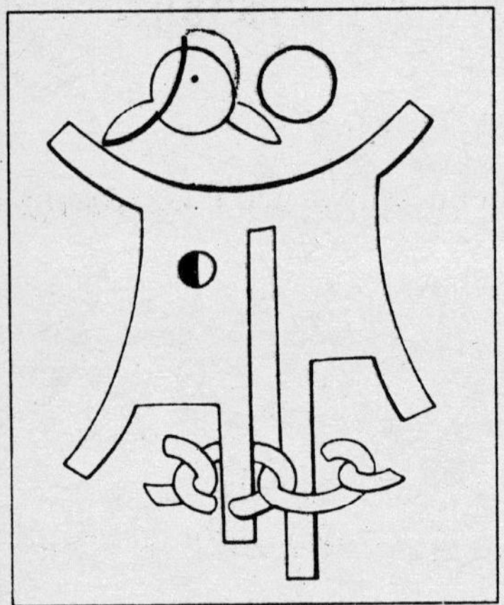

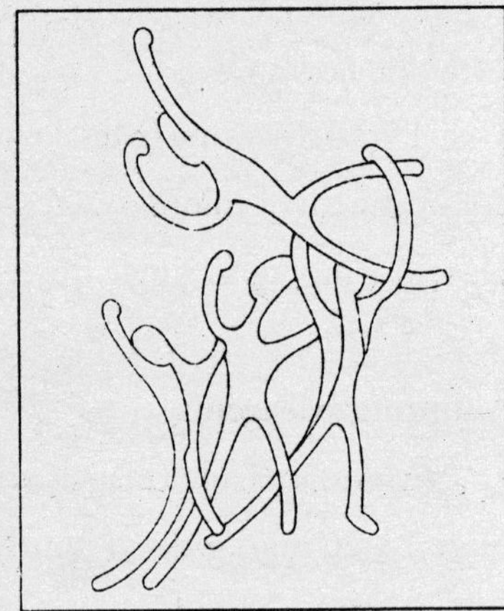

Section Three

To Train an Early Brain

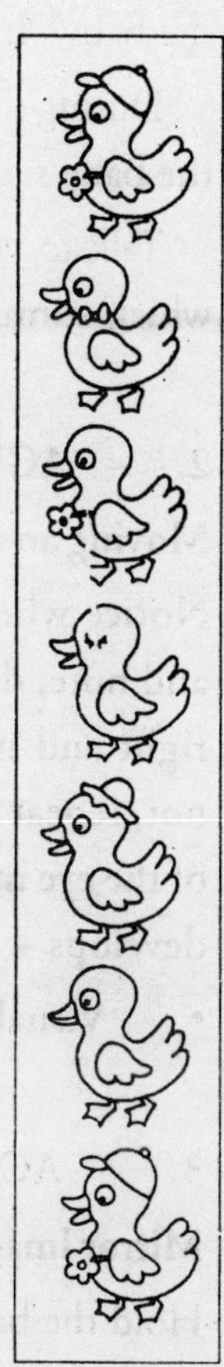

A child starts learning since birth. Brain development is much more vulnerable to environmental influence. Environment affects the number of brain cells and connections among them. Children not exposed to inadequate amount of play and touching develop 20-30% smaller brain than normal.

What is a developing brain?

Scientists have confirmed that babies are born with billions of brain cells, much more than they have at the age of three and twice as many as they have as an adult. Growing his basic skills at the right time is essential to maximize a child's learning process.

Are repeating activities more helpful to a child?

Yes, repeating activities are more advantageous. More a baby repeats an act, the more secure and responsive he will be. Repetitive activities will improve the infant's thinking and reasoning. Child should be nurtured with love and gentleness.

1. AGE 0 – WEEK 1

Move the body parts

Observe the baby's hand movements. Test his grasp. Put the baby's left and right palms together. It will help to develop a feeling of awareness of both sides of his body.

Observe the baby's leg and foot movements. Touch and hold the baby's left and right foot and note the baby's reaction.

During this week, please observe your baby's movements. Wrap the baby securely in a blanket during the first week of life.

Talk to your baby. Sing or hum to him. You may play a CD which stimulates the baby's sense of hearing.

2. AGE 0 – WEEK 3

Moving an object

Notice whether the baby fixes his eyes on you. Hold a rattle and note, does the baby look at it. Move the rattle from left to right and note if his eyes follow from left to right or not. If not, repeat it after some days off and on. This is the beginning of the eye movement training required for reading. This activity develops –

- Visual stimulation of moving objects.

3. AGE 0 – WEEK 5

Mirror Image

Hold the baby close enough to look at himself in a large mirror. Does the baby smile or coo? Talk to the baby and call him by his name.

- This will develop the baby's awareness of his own image.
- It will develop his listening skills.

4. AGE 0 – WEEK 7

Response to noise

Make a sound with a bell. Note, does the baby turn his head, eyes or body in the direction of the sound? Hold the bell in front of the baby, does he reach for the bell?

This activity develops –

- The baby's listening awareness.

5. AGE 0 – WEEK 11

Eye-Hand Coordination

Lay the baby on his back. Put a multicoloured soft ball on the baby's stomach. Roll the ball up to his chest and neck. Watch the baby's eyes and hand. Does he reach for the ball and respond?

This activity helps in –

- Tactile sensation that stimulates the baby to hold the object.
- Develops focussing on object.

6. AGE 0 – WEEK 18

Nursery Rhymes

Read and sing rhymes for the baby. Repeat each one several times. Words of rhymes will be liked by the baby.

Activity develops –

- Listening skills
- Language enrichment

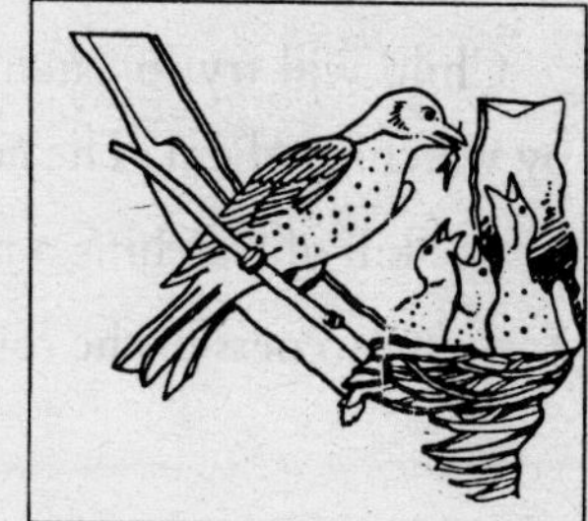

7. AGE 0 – WEEK 20

Awareness of hands

Move your hands apart and then bring them together again. Repeat this on many occasions in front of the eyes of the baby. The baby should enjoy this .

This activity develops –

- Awareness of hands.
- Listening skills.

8. AGE 0 – WEEK 35

Water Splash

During bath, make a splashing sound with the water. Exaggerating the sound will attract the baby's attention.

This activity develops –

- Listening for different sounds.
- Awareness of wetness.

9. AGE 0 – WEEK 38

Blowing Bubbles

Buy a jar of bubble blowing solution. Blow colourful bubbles to entertain the baby. Then try to catch the bubbles.

Child will try to catch the bubbles too. He will be delighted by watching them. The activity will develop –

- Skill of watching a moving object.
- Awareness of the round shape of bubbles.

10. AGE 0 – WEEK 42

Coloured Squares

Take 12 squares of cardboard of equal size having a different design. Two squares should be similar so there will be six sets of two each.

Observe which of the squares attracts the baby's attention. Encourage the baby to feel and touch.

When the baby becomes more familiar he may show an interest in matching them.

The activity develops –

- Awareness of different colours.
- Awareness of the square shape.
- The art of matching squares.

11. AGE 0 – WEEK 45

Dropping an article in a container

Take a container having a circular hole in the lid. Give the baby a spoon and encourage him to put in the hole. He may need a little help at first but with several attempts he should meet success. The activity can be used later for baby to do independently.

The activity develops –

- Eye-hand coordination.
- Skill in putting articles into holes.
- Develops confidence.

12. AGE 0 – WEEK 50

Recognising parts of the face

Throughout and whenever possible, stress up on the parts of the face. If the child is confused, spend several days on the eyes, then progress and spend many days on, the nose, mouth, ears and hair. When the baby becomes confident, encourage him to point to or touch a part of face on request.

This activity develops

- Listening skills.
- Awareness of parts of face.
- Skill in associating different parts of face with their names.

Age One to Two Years

Although a child becomes a little bit independent at this age but he still needs guidance. Try to understand your baby by noting his daily pattern of behaviour. A child of this age has a very short span of attention.

During this period songs and rhymes will capture the child's interest. Continue to repeat them often. A child at this age is curious and will explore his environment by pulling, pushing and poking and will remain very busy. He will show more affection and will use gestures or point to convey wishes. The more you interact with him, talking, playing, hugging and kissing, the more comfortable your child will be with you.

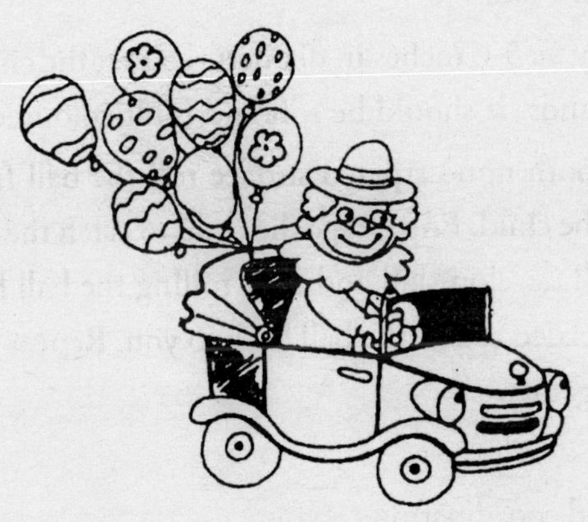

AGE 1 YEAR – WEEK 2

Spools

Encourage the child to bring two spools together. Sing the words "one, two, and two." You and your child can have fun rolling a spool back and forth to each other. Show the child how to put one spool over other and encourage him to try independently. Help him if needed and praise him for any positive action.

Activity develops –

- Awareness of sets of two.
- Awareness of the pattern of 1-2.
- Free exploration.

AGE 1 YEAR – WEEK 5

Playing with a ball

The ball may be 5-6 inches in diametre so that the child can hold it in both hands. It should be soft and multicoloured.

On a smooth non-carpeted surface roll the ball from a short distance to the child. Encourage the child to catch the ball. Slowly the child will develop skill and start rolling the ball back. Much practice is needed to roll the ball back to you. Repeat this activity for weeks together.

This activity develops –

- Hand coordination.
- Tactile sensation.
- Following directions.

AGE 1 YEAR – WEEK 8

Walking on a straight line

Draw a 5 feet long straight line on the floor. First you walk on the designated straight line while the child watches you. Then persue the child to walk on the line. Praise the child even if he fails. Repeat this activity at least for 2 weeks. Child will slowly become confident.

This activity develops –

- Concentration
- Legs, foot and eye co-ordination
- Following direction.

AGE 1 YEAR – WEEK 12

Exposure to outside garden

Go outside to a garden. Look at the grass and tell the child about its colour. Allow the child to touch the grass. He may pick up some blades of it.

Show the child the multicoloured flowers. Child may be allowed to smell the flowers.

Then introduce him to trees too. At home read about and see pictures of trees, grass and flowers.

This activity develops –

- Awareness of different colours.
- Vocabulary enrichment.
- Awareness about garden.

Exploring with water

Allow the child to play with water and sponge. He may be allowed to have a feel of the sponge before putting it in water and afterwards too. Encourage the child to listen for sounds that the water produces when it is splashed.

This activity develops –

- Eye-hand co-ordination.
- Awareness of sense of touch.
- Observation skills.

AGE 1 YEAR – WEEK 18

Putting keys through a slit hole

Collect 10 keys and a container having a slit through which keys can be pushed through. Encourage the child to pick up a key and push it through the slit.

This activity develops –

- Fine motor control.
- Following direction.
- Eye-hand co-ordination.

AGE 1 YEAR – WEEK 23

Climbing up and downstairs.

This is a good age for the child to practice up and down the climbing stairs. He may be allowed to climb 4 stairs only at a time.

As the child is encouraged to go up and down the stairs it will become more interesting for him. All this should be practiced under supervision. Once he develops confidence he will enjoy going up and down the stairs over and over again.

The activity will result in –

- Awareness of 'up' and 'down'.
- Gross motor co-ordination.
- Self-confidence.

AGE 1 YEAR – WEEK 28

Cardboard puzzle

The picture on the cardboard may be of a simple and known object like a butterfly, house or a dog etc. Start by dividing the picture into two pieces only.

First show the child a complete picture, then mix up the pieces. Now encourage the child to put the card pieces back correctly. Help the child if he does not understand. Encourage him. Use one puzzle at a time. Picture should be a large and colourful one with little detail. Too many pieces will confuse the child.

This activity helps in –

- Developing awareness that two parts make a whole.
- More awareness of colours.

AGE 1 YEAR – WEEK 30

Carrying a tray

Select an unbreakable tray and put light, non breakable objects on it. Now encourage the child to balance the tray and carry it a short distance. The tray should not be big. Praise the child as he carries the tray. Remind the child to walk slowly.

This activity will develop –

- Skill with the sense of balance.
- Coordination of both hands.

AGE 1 YEAR – WEEK 32

Recognising the room

Take the hand of the child in your hand and ask him to take you to his room. Then walk to the bathroom and identify it.

Praise the child if this command is followed correctly. If the child seems confused make him understand the correct recognition of room and bathroom.

Continue this activity with your bathroom and bedroom. It may take several days for the child to go to the correct room.

This activity develops

- Awareness of rooms and their position.
- Following directions.
- Confidence.

AGE 1 YEAR – WEEK 36

Walking on stepping stones

Take a child to a garden where a footpath has different sizes of stones to walk on leaving a small green space between two stones.

The child may be asked to step on stones only placed at a specific distance. He may be asked not to put his foot in between the gap of the two stones.

This activity will develop –

- Better co-ordination of large and small muscles.
- Increased awareness of big and small objects.
- An awareness of distance.

AGE 1 YEAR – WEEK 46

Pouring water from one container to another

Train the child to transfer water from one cup to another. Show and tell the child that one of the containers is empty and the others one is full. This will serve to enrich the child's awareness of these two concepts.

This activity develops –

- Observation skill.
- Awareness of empty and full.
- Eye-hand cordination.

AGE 1 YEAR – WEEK 50

Button and zip

Train the child to button and unbutton his coat. Button should be of large size so that the child may catch hold of it easily.

If he is able to do this within 2 weeks, the child should be free to open and fasten a zip.

The activity develops –

- An awareness of fastening clothes.
- Confidence and independence.
- Eye-hand coordination.

AGE 1 YEAR – WEEK 52

Open and close the door

You open the door and close it in front of the child. See that the door knob is easily accessible. Allow the child to practice turning the knob. The child will be interested and may enjoy exploring it independently. Or another occasion open and close a door in another room. The child should be allowed to open and close different types of doors.

Child will develop –

- Skill in turning knobs to open and close a door.
- An awareness of the concepts of 'open' and 'close'.
- Confidence.

AGE 1 YEAR – WEEK 52

Hide and Seek

Encourage the child to cover his eyes with his hands and when you are hidden say 'Find me'. Hopefully, the child can find you behind a sofa or a curtain. The child may find you by following your voice. Do this several times. When the child becomes confident, hide at a different place.

Next time ask the child to hide. Note that whether the child selects the same places or somewhere new. Finding a new hiding place shows that he has picked up the game. But if he selects the old places only, he may be asked and encouraged to find a new place to hide. Two-three children can also play this game under the guidance of an adult person.

The activity develops –

- Skill in tracing the sound of a person's voice.
- Awareness of 'out of sight'.
- Listening for a purpose.
- Confidence.

Two – Three Years

Now the child is much more active as well as inquisitive. He recognises size, colour and shapes well.

He can talk and recite short rhymes. Now he can remember events sequentially.

The child will like to draw strange figures if a pencil is given to him. First he draws up and down. Soon he starts making strokes from left to right and in a circular fashion.

Many children of this age like jumping, running, kicking, dancing, pushing and pulling. A child has developed bette· motor coordination by now. At this time fine motor activities should be encouraged.

The child can easily identify the members of his family. He may even be able to tell his name.

He will love to listen to fantasy stories from his grandmother. He will imitate many words and sounds.

AGE 2 YEARS – WEEK 6

Walking with a box

Take 2 boxes which will fit the child's feet well. Let the child be helped to put one foot in each box. Now encourage him to walk with the boxes on, touch a door at a distance and come back to you.

The child may also enjoy sliding the boxes.

This activity develops –

- Gross motor co-ordination.
- Awareness of completing a task.
- Pleasure of doing something new.

AGE 2 YEARS – WEEK 12

Recognising members of the family

Show a family photo to the child and point out each member of the family by name. Talk about members in detail so that the child may remember. Use the words father, mother, dada, dadi, brother etc.

This exercise may be repeated for a week.

The advantage of this exercise is –

- More awareness of family.
- Recognition of members of the family.

AGE 2 YEARS – WEEK 14

Painting

Protect the child's clothes and make him year a sleeveless vest. Give water colours, a brush and a drawing sheet.

Show the child how to dip and rub the brush against the sides of the bottles to avoid excess paint.

Now ask the child to paint the paper within the frame boundary already drawn. Nowadays many such books are available in the

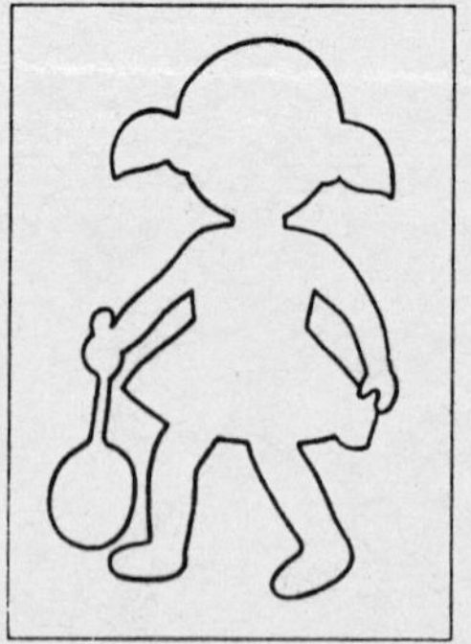

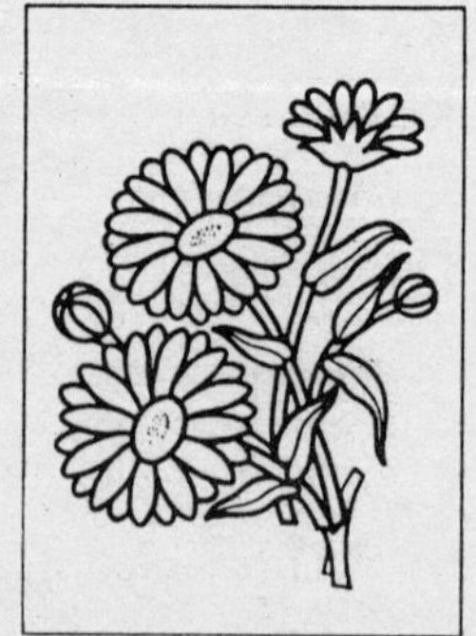

market to colour the figures. Observe the child's strokes. Tell him a story about the picture.

Activity develops –

- Creativity.
- Free exploration and recognition of colours.
- Eye, hand and arm co-ordination.

AGE 2 YEARS – WEEK 15

Animals

Use pictures with minimal details of each animal. With each picture tell him the name of the animal. Repeat till you are sure that he can recognise correctly. Select the common animals like dog, horse, cat, donkey, cow, pig, elephant, etc. You can show the child these animals in real life too.

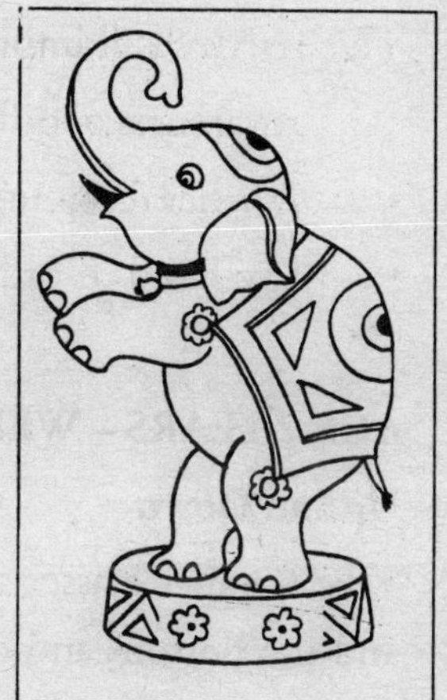

This will develop –

- The skill of recognising animals.
- Memory recall.
- Confidence.
- Listening skills.

AGE 2 YEARS – WEEK 18

Putting articles on a line

Draw a metre long line on the ground. Give the child some articles such as a block, keys, football, a spool etc.

Ask the child to put these articles on the line. Then encourage the child to pick them up. Repeat the activity on different occasions with different objects on each occasion.

This activity will develop –

- Awareness of putting objects on a line.
- Recognising the objects.

AGE 2 YEARS – WEEK 20

Outline the shape

Introduce the child with different shapes of coloured cardboard. Let him identify the circle, square, triangle and rectangle. Each of these must have a different colour too. Repeat the process on many occasions.

This activity will improve –

- Awareness of different shapes.
- Further recognition of colours.
- Eye-hand co-ordination.

AGE 2 YEARS – WEEK 24

Up and Down

Take 6 paper glasses and 6 paper cups. Show the child the top and the bottom and of the glasses. Begin by placing the first 2 glasses, one facing up and another facing down. Encourage the child to put the other 4 glasses similarly.

In the next row ask him to put the cups similarly. When the child understands the game, different commands of alternate cup and glass may be given.

This activity helps –

- An awareness of 'up' and 'down'.
- Fine and gross motor action.
- Free exploration and problem solving.

AGE 2 YEARS – WEEK 32

Ladder Walk

A wooden ladder can be laid flat on the floor. Show the child how to walk in the gaps. Once he is able to do so and has reached the other end, tell the child to turn around and come back. Repeat this for a week.

This activity develops –

- Awareness of the concept of 'in-between'.
- Coarse motor coordination.
- Body balance.
- Listening and following directions.

AGE 2 YEARS – WEEK 38

Putting eggs in a row

Ask the child to put coloured eggs (rubber/plastic ones) one in each cup. Then ask him to put eggs of one colour in one row and eggs of another colour in the next row.

This activity develops –

- An understanding of rows.
- Indenpendence.
- Confidence.

AGE 2 YEARS – WEEK 42

Different fruits

Collect one each of a mango, orange, banana, apple, peach, papaya and pineapple. Show one fruit at a time and tell its name. Then introduce the other fruits one by one. Tell characteristics of each fruit.

Then ask the child to pick up a fruit by its name. Continue this till you are satisfied that he collects a correct fruit. Later on taste him the name of each fruit one by one.

This acvitity may be done many times with different fruits and vegetables.

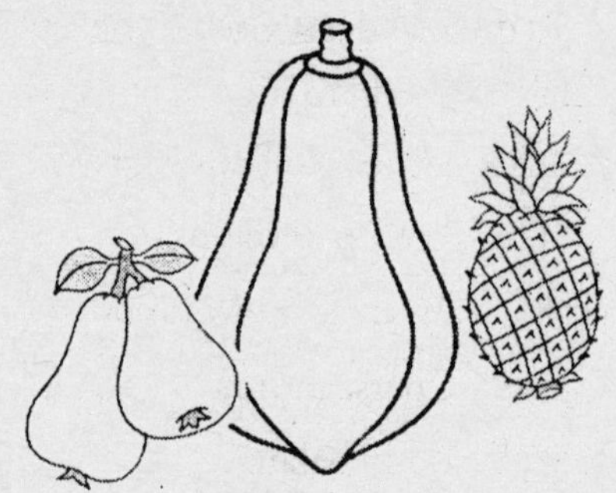

Activity develops –

- Awareness of shape and size of fruits.
- Listening skills.
- Confidence.

AGE 2 YEARS – WEEK 44

Hot and Cold

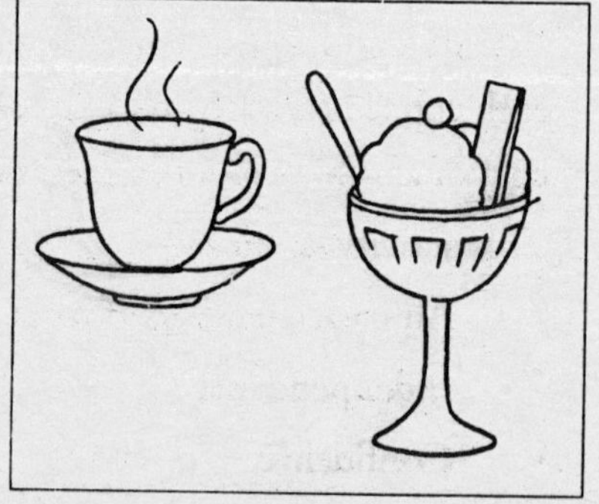

Take a cup of hot coffee and a cup of ice cream. Let him touch the steaming coffee cup and the cold ice scream. Keep watch so that he does not burn himself. Tell the child that the ice cream is cold and allow him to touch it again and do the same with the coffee.

At each meal, discuss which foods are hot and which are cold.

This activity develops –

- Awareness of hot and cold.
- Art of differentiating 'hot and cold'.

AGE 2 YEARS – WEEK 48

Throwing a ball

Allow a child to throw a ball. Note how much distance the ball has covered. Then ask him again to throw the ball from the same point and collect the ball. Play this game in a garden or an open place.

This activity develops –

- Gross motor co-ordination.
- Awareness of distance.
- Eye-hand co-ordination.

AGE 2 YEARS – WEEK 50

Utility items

Assemble various household items, e.g. one each of a spoon, book, shoe, tooth brush etc. Talk about each item, then tell the child

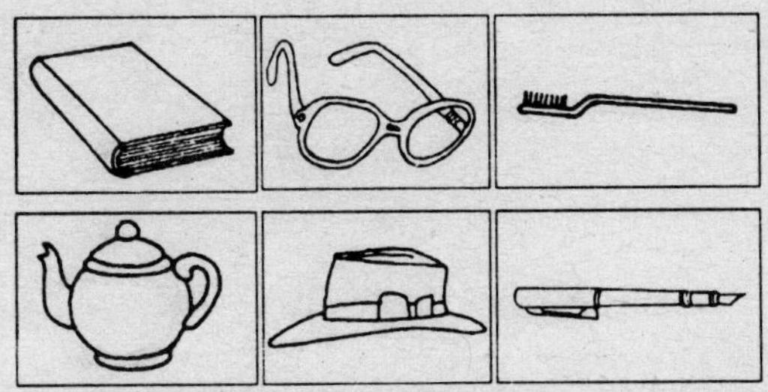

about its utility. Ask him to recognise each item. Assist the child if he needs help.

This activity will develop –

- Language enrichment.
- Awareness of objects of purpose.
- Observational skills.

AGE 2 YEARS – WEEK 52

Foot pushing

In an open space ask the child to push a football. Ask him not to kick the ball but to push it slowly.

When the child has developed some co-ordination ask him to take the ball to the designated area by pushing it with his foot.

This activity develops

- Eye-foot coordination.
- Reaching a goal.

Age Three to Four Years

During this periods child is more self-centred. He shows the signs of more independence. He has already picked up more words.

He develops interest in fine motor activities and has already developed better small muscle coordination.

Stories, rhymes, songs become a part of his life. He may count up to 50 or 100. He becomes very inquisitive.

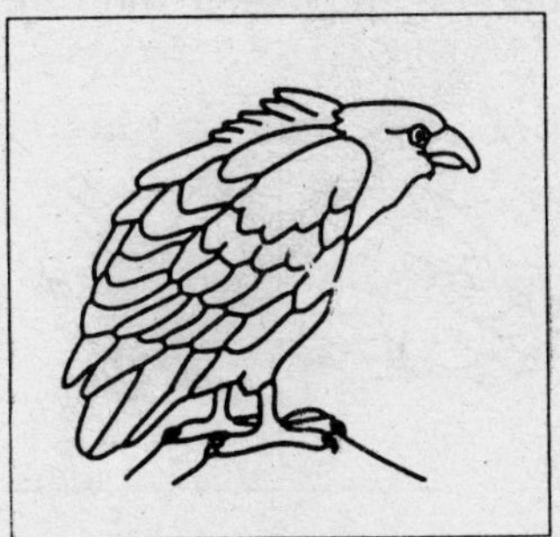

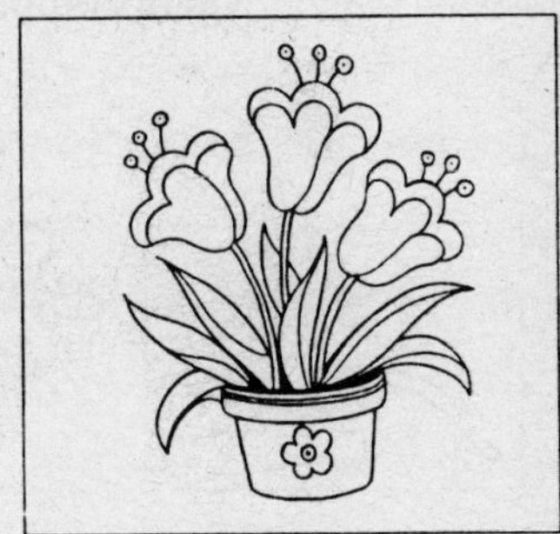

AGE 3 YEARS – WEEK 2

Bouncing of ball

Choose a ball of 6-8" diametre which bounces well. A smaller ball will be difficult to catch.

Show the child how to drop the ball and catch it after it bounces. Allow the child to hold the ball, drop it, watch it bouncing and attempt to catch it. Stand behind the child and help him to catch the bouncing ball. Count how many times the child can bounce and catch the ball without missing. The child can throw the ball against a wall and then hold it.

This activity develops –

- Eye-hand co-ordination.
- Skill in throwing and catching a ball.
- Awareness of 'up' and 'down'.

AGE 3 YEARS – WEEK 4

Recognition of animals

Show him a picture of a frog and tell him it has four limbs and that a frog moves by hopping and jumping. If possible show him

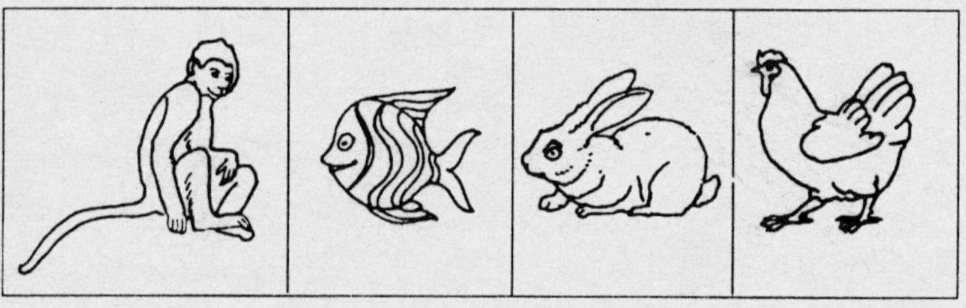

how a frog hops around.

Then show him a picture of a bird and tell him about its features.

Later on you may tell him about a fish. Tell him that it lives in water and has no hands and feet. Show him the birds of different kinds also.

This activity develops –

- Awareness of different kinds of animals.
- Language enrichment.
- Keen sense of observation.

AGE 3 YEARS – WEEK 8

Climb up and down

Lay down a small ladder against a stable object so that it may not slip down.

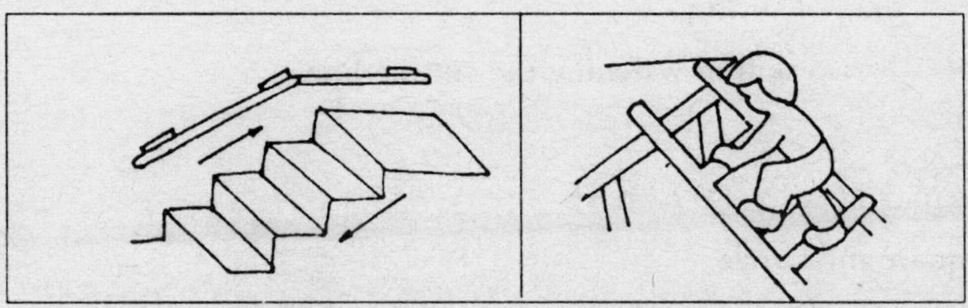

Ask the child to climb up and down the ladder. A child of this age likes to climb, slide, run or skip. But keep a watch so that he does not slip down and hurt himself.

This activity helps in –

- Developing the concept of up and down.
- Develops eye-hand-foot co-ordination.
- Develops gross motor skill.
- Develops confidence.

AGE 3 YEARS – WEEK 12

Use of Scissors

Scissors have to be used carefully. They should be blunt and not very pointed. Show the child how to hold a pair of scissors. Tell him that the thumb should always be up. Then ask

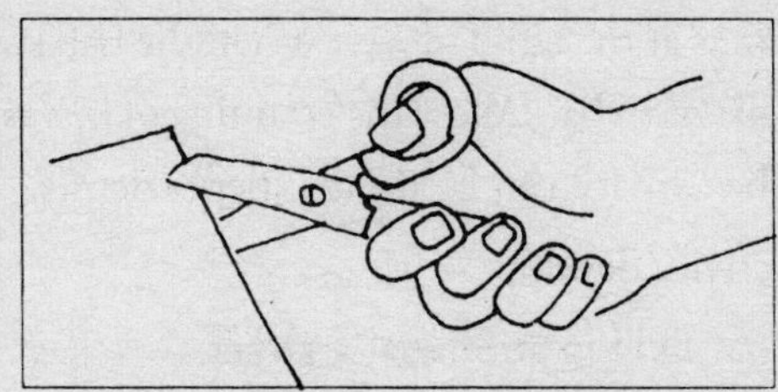

him to cut a paper. Later on draw a line bisecting the paper and ask him to cut along the line. Ask him to do this repeatedly. Continue to draw lines for the child to cut.

Activity will develop –

- Skill of cutting.
- Visual skill in watching the cutting line.

AGE 3 YEARS – WEEK 16

Square and Circle

Show the child how to draw a circle. You may show him by tracing a circle around a tea plate. Ask him to do so as well. His pencil may slip off and on.

Similarly you can ask him to draw a square. Continue to play till the child is able to draw successfully.

Child will develop –

- More awareness of circle and squre.
- Eye-hand co-ordination.
- Confidence.

AGE 3 YEARS – WEEK 16

Hit and Miss

Suspend a ball. The string should be long enough so that the ball hangs at the child's level. When the ball swings ask him to hit the ball with a bat. Allow the counting of hits as long as he is interested. The activity can be done independently.

Activity develops –

- Skill in aiming at a target.

- Eye-arm co-ordination.
- Skill in anticipating the return.

AGE 3 YEARS – WEEK 20

Nuts and Bolts

Assemble different sizes of metal nuts and bolts. Show the child how to thread nuts and bolts.

If the child has problems with the nuts and the bolt help him. The child can sort the nuts and bolts according to size to try and thread them later on. He will require guidance off and on.

This activity helps in –

- Matching the skills.
- Eye-hand co-ordination.
- Problem solving skills.

AGE YEARS 3 – WEEK 24

Pouring Water

Take a big plastic jar full of water and put 6 plastic glasses of different colours in a line.

Allow the child to hold the jar of water and tell him to fill the glasses one by one.

Throughout the process you should talk to your child. If he spills some water do not scold him.

Child will develop –

- Skill of pouring a liquid.
- Awareness of empty and full.

- Observation of skill.
- Confidence.

AGE 3 YEARS – WEEK 34

Taste

Assemble some sugar, salt, lime and peeper.

Make a child taste these articles and explain the different tastes

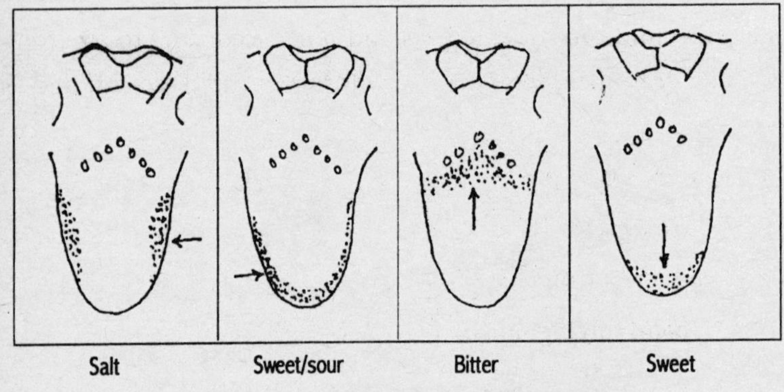

POSITION OF TASTE BUDS ON A HUMAN TONGUE

to him. Emphasize the four words 'sweet' 'salty' 'bitter' and 'sour'. During this time you can talk about cake, pickles etc.

This activity will develop –

- Mind and visual co-ordination.
- Skill in recognising different tastes.

AGE 3 YEARS – WEEK 42

Folding of paper

Cut out one circle and a few squares of paper measuring 8-10 inches. Put a line with a marker across the middle of one square and diagonally in another.

Show the line across the square and ask the child to fold the square along that line; similarly ask him to fold the circle.

Allow the child to fold the papers again and again. Refolding will be an interesting fun.

This activity develops –

- More awareness of basic shapes.
- Eye-hand co-ordination in folding.
- Confidence.

AGE 3 YEARS – WEEK 52

Junk box

Allow the child to collect many simple items. Some items may be of interest to a child like plastic flowers, small car, keys, spools, comb etc.

Keep the box of junk indefinately because certain children keep themselves busy in examining and experimenting with such items. These items should be safe and not pointed.

The activity develops –

- Freedom of choice.
- Independence and freedom.

Age Four to Five

By now the child has grown up socially, physically and mentally. Now he requires friends to play and for proper development. It will broaden his outlook in life. Children learn from each other. At this age a child starts reading and seeing pictures in a book.

Coordination of hand skills is much improved by this age. The child can be taught writing ABCD.

AGE 4 YEARS – WEEK 1

Numbers

Every week tell him about numbers, like in the first week let him know the number (1)

Second week the number [2]

Third week the number [3]

Fourth week the number [4]

Fifth week the number [5]

Sixth week the number [6]

Seventh week number [7]

Eighth week number [8]

Ninth week number [9]

Tenth week number [10]

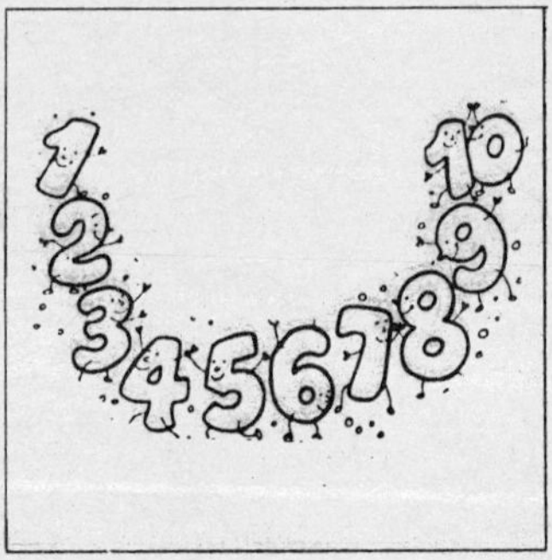

Every week the child should learn to recognise one extra number and if possible one should persuade him to overwrite on a dotted figure.

AGE 4 YEARS – WEEK 14

Alphabet

Every week introduce him to one alphabet of the English language A to Z.

A	B	C	D	E
F	G	H	I	J
K	L	M	N	O
P	Q	R	S	T
U	V	W	X	Y
Z				

Side by side child should be taught his mother tongue. Parents have to teach him simple manners before he goes to school. He has to be told stories off and on to improve his knowledge.

Your Child and Zodiac Signs

Mani Raj Sharma

In todays fast changing world, every body still longs to know what the future hold. Every body is deeply concerned about tomorrow. Modern science has confirmed some of astrology foundations unintentionally and some of it reluctantly.

There are 12 zodiac signs and sun spends about one month in each. Motion of sun is regular and meaningful predictions are possible which every parent wants to know about his son/ daughter.

ARIES CHILD (March 21 to April 20)

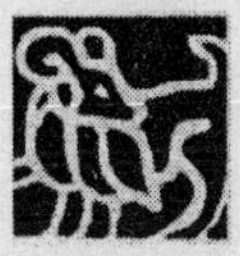

He is often quite strong and enthusiastic. He is not easily discouraged by temporary set backs. He is natural born leader. You cannot stop him when he is exploring. He will like extra curricural activities. He has enthusiasm. He does not want only traditional things. He is courageous, optimistic and friendly. He remains busy to succeed one way or the other.

Boys They seek adventure having high energy levels. They will shirk taking a risk. They are fond of shopping. They are not selfish. They love relationship and will like to break its shackles. They make sensible talk.

Girls Take care of their temper tantrums. They calm down soon after little assurance. They are extremely affectionate and become friend for life long.

TAURUS CHILD (April 21 to May 21)

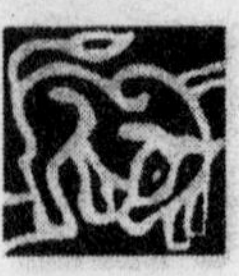

These persons are known for their ability to concentrate and for their tenacity. He gets very well with others. He never leaves anything unfinished. He is strong and healthy. He is methodical and dependable. He wants secure and stable environment at home. He is not fond of surprises.

Boys They do not take risk. They have fixed play and meal time. Their attitude will be an artistic. They make a good company. They tolerate challanges. As a friend they are dependable. They don't like stringiness. They like fun. They are fond of art and beauty in all forms. Still they are realistic. They value consistency in their lives.

Girls She is very fond of good clothes and food. She is fond of toys and kitchen tools. She has lovely singing voice. She is reliable, loyal and understanding. She may not make friends easily.

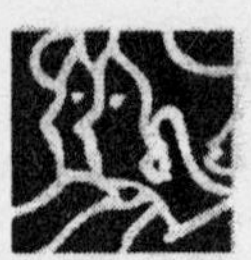

GEMINI (May 22 to June 21)

He is bright and quick witted, some of them are capable of doing many different things. He keeps an open mind and remains anxious to learn new things. He is likely to be happy and lively child. He is very active, hence it is very difficult to control him. He is always full of fresh move. He lives in a dual world of fantasy and reality. Some Geminions are sharp tongued.

Boys He is fond of adventures and travelling. He lacks patience. He constantly needs new interests. He can achieve his goals. He is governed by brain and not by heart. He can understand both sides of problem. He is an adoptable person and can make himself at home almost anywhere.

Girls She is an adaptable making herself at home almost anywhere. The Geminian is quite charming. A good talker, she often is the centre of attraction at any gathering. She is kind and loves nature. She is eager and bright. She is bold and have some musculine features. She enjoys outdoor games.

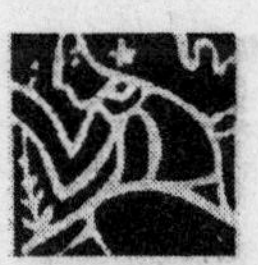

VIRGO CHILD (August 22 to September 22)

He is a busy person and a good planner. He is practical and not afraid of hard work. He knows how to attain what he desires. He never shirks his duties. He wants to do every thing with perfection. Such people are successful in life. He makes good critics.

Boys He is sensitive about how others feel. He has no trouble in expressing himself. He is a constructive child. He wants to do every thing himself. On occasions he may become emotionless and cool.

Girls Such girl gives more importance to her looks. She will adhere the moderate way of life. She does not like work done by others. She is plain spoken and down to earth. She may be interested in art and literature. She is very observant and never secretive. She is too neat and tidy.

CANCERIAN CHILD (June 21 to July 20)

He is of understanding nature. He is loving and sympathetic person. He will not hurt any one. These children have emotional feelings with their surroundings. They evaluate every one and every thing in term of feelings. They are hypersensitive and loves quiet and secure environment. They hate to see sufferings of others and will do what they can do to help others.

Boys On occasions these are moody. Such boys offer love, affection and warmth to their caretakers. They have fluctuation in his temper. They enjoy being surrounded by familiar things and people they loves.

Girls She is kind and loves nature. She will like to learn everything. The cancer woman often is given to crying when the smallest thing goes wrong.

She has much more love and emotional warmth. She aspects the same from others. She does not make many friends and is governed by heart than brain.

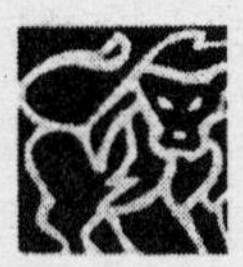

LEO CHILD (July 21 to August 21)

They seems to be good organisers and administrators. They are overflowing with sympathy and are generous to a fault. They defend their friends. They are lucky in money matters. They are fond of welcoming people to their house and entertaining them.

Boys He has plenty of confidence and can share his toys. He is generous. He has plenty of energy and drive. He has a quick mind. He believes that only he is capable of doing things well. On occasions he may be rude, otherwise a loving child.

Girls She is reliable and friendly. She is kind and confident. She is a good host and confident. She gets whatever she wants. She means what she says. She is never unsure of herself. She is an ambitious.

LIBRA CHILD (September 23 to October 22)

They love harmony. They admire beauty and grace. They are loyal and amiable. They are against unjustice. Many of them are escapists. They have great fore sight and intution. Their first impression comes to true.

Boys They are often successful. They are good in studies. They reach on top in their respective branch.

Girls In married life they are seldom happy. They crave for peace and happiness of home life. In friend circle they are largely saught after as companions. They enjoy possessions and luxuries. They have a keen sense of beauty. They like handsome furnishings and clothes, being artistically inclined.

SCORPIO CHILD (October 23 to November 20)

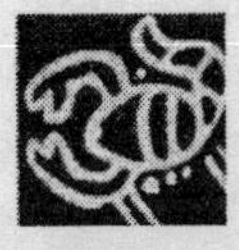

They have clever idea in business and politics and are best advisers. They generally leave things for tomorrow. They are mental fighters and most subtle in agreements. They have strong personalities. They are easily attracted towards opposite sex. They are brave and courageous. Obstacles don't frighten them.

Boys He has strong will power. He is quite tender and loving. He is sincere and. he never utters anything which he does not mean. He sets a goal for himself and achieves it in a direct way. He is a determined child.

Girls She is quite tender and loving. She believes sincerity in all relationship. She sticks to her principals. On occasions she proves hypersensitive. She may take more interest in sexual activities. She knows what she wants out of life. She is a positive child.

SAGITTARIUS (November 23 to December 20)

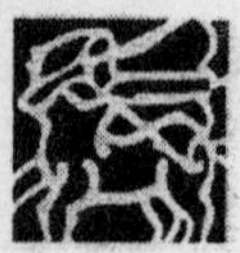

These are often honest and forth right. Their approach to life is earnest and open. They are broad minded and tolerant. Their standards are high. They cut good jokes and are keen on fun which makes them very popular with others.

Boys He is a lively person who enjoys sports and outdoor life. he is fond of pets and animals. He is not selfish or proudy. He is seldom critical and is almost generous. They mismanage their finances. They may be honest at the wrong time. Some boys may prove undisciplined wasting a lot of energy.

Girls They are great workers. They resent deception. They are religious by nature. They love music. They may marry on impulse and later on may regret. They love to make their husband successful and will sacrifice everything to that end. They make best of mother. They like to be independent.

CAPRICORN CHILD (December 22 to January 20)

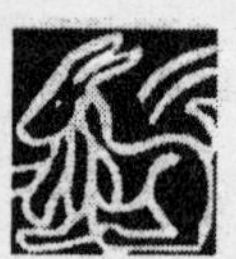

Child is really a go getter type. Child is capable of tackling many tasks at a time. Child will help you in kitchen. He will like to behave an adult man. He wants complete power. He recognises reliability. Such child do not want change in routine. He does not take risk. He makes very few friends.

Boys He is a hard worker and remains busy in making plans. He is practical and reliable. His interest in material things may be exaggerated on occasion. Still he is a trust worthy boy.

Girls These are studious and hard working, may be topper in class. They are friendly and conservative by nature.

AQUARIUS CHILD (January 21 to February 19)

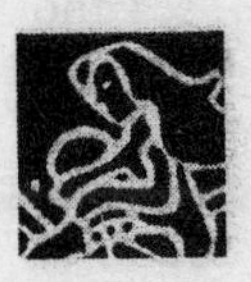

He is very honest and forthright. His standards for himself are very high. He can always be relied upon. He is forgetful and remain dreamy. He proves to be unpredictable. He will not follow set routine. He wants to remain independent and fight for a cause. He does not like loneliness.

Boys He is most tolerant. He is like philospher and wants to chase even wind. He wants to know the cause of an every event. He obeys mother. He is a good judge to know reality and cannot tolerate his trust being broken.

Girls These are quiet and don't cause tension to others. Unspoken tension can deeply disturb them. She likes to be of service to others.

PISCES CHILD (February 19 to March 20)

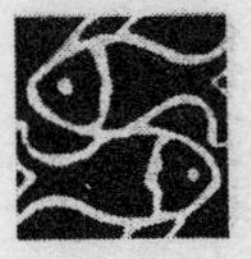

He is of sympathetic nature and helps others. He is broadminded and does not criticise others. He accepts people as a whole. He is trust worthy and loyal. Some pisces may be depressed and feel that the world is a cold and cruel place. Some may be lazy. His will power may be low.

Boys He believes in helping each other. He cooperates others and tries to adjust others. He has a strong intuitive sense. He is loyal to his friends. He is easily discouraged.

Girls She lets things happen without giving the least bit of resistance. In matter of sex she can rather be permissive. In family she is willing to do more than her share. The sick and troubled members often turn to her for advice and assistance. She is loyal and generous in money matters. She is generally fond of sea and rivers. She will make a successful lady.

Baby Record of Birth

Date ____________ Time ________

Place ____________

Colour of eyes ____________________

Colour of hair ____________________

Complexion ____________________

Weight ____________________

Length ____ ____________________

Circumference of head ____________

Birth mark if any ____________

How does the baby look____________

Zodiac sign ____________________

Blood group ____________________

Delivery Normal/Forcep/Caesarian

____

____

____

	FATHER	MOTHER
Full name		
Place of birth		
Date of birth		
Education		
Qualification		
Date of marriage		
Place of marriage		
Hobbies		
Blood group		

RELATIVES	DATE OF BIRTH
Paternal Grandfather	
Paternal Grandmother	
Maternal Grandfather	
Maternal Grandmother	
Uncle	
Aunty	
Brother	
Sister	
Cousins	

VACCINATION

• Tripple Vaccine Date

1st injection ____________________

2nd injection ____________________

3rd injection ____________________

• Measles ________ ________ ________

• Chicken pox ________ ________ ________

• Polio ________ ________ ________

________ ________ ________

________ ________ ________

Booster doses

HEIGHT/WEIGHT RECORD

	Height (cms)	Weight (kg)
Birth		
First Month		
Second "		
Third "		
Fourth "		
Fifth "		
Sixth "		
Eight "		
Tenth "		
Twentieth "		
2 years		
3 years		
4 years		
5 years		

Appearance of teeth	Date	Teeth	Date

RECORD OF THE CHILD'S DEVELOPMENT

Birth to 6 Months Development	Date of Notice
1. Responds to sound	
2. Responds to light	
3. Turns head side to side	
4. Smiles	
5. Legs are extended	
6. Plays with hands	
7. Plays with feet	
8. Enjoys looking in the mirror	
9. Attempts to grasp moving things	
10. Sits alone	

If 5 or fewer parametres achieved	Delayed
If 7 "	Slightly delayed
If 8 to 10	Satisfactory development

7th to 12th Months Development	Date of Notice
1. Rolls over	
2. Transfers objects hand to hand	
3. Creeps/crawls	
4. Drops objects & tries to pick up	
5. Responds by name	
6. Pushes objects to make way	
7. Pulls up to standing position	
8. Walks holding furniture	
9. Says Mama/Dada	
10. Walks a few steps	

5 Parametres achieved	Delayed development
7 "	Slightly delayed
8 to 10 "	Satisfactory

1–2 Years Development	Date of Notice
1. Crawls up stairs	
2. Follows simple directions	
3. Names familiar objects	
4. Explores drawers	
5. Listens to stories	
6. Kicks a ball	
7. Walks backwards	
8. Runs	
9. Helps in domestic tasks	
10. Plays simple games	

5 Parameters achieved	Delayed development
7 "	Slightly delayed "
8 to 10 "	Satisfactory "

2–3 Years Development	Date of Notice
1. Opens and closes door	
2. Enjoys climbing	
3. Walks down one step	
4. Helps in dressing/ undressing	
5. Jumping from higher to lower level	
6. Knows full name	
7. Knows his sex	
8. Imitates actions/sounds	
9. Participate in active games	
10. Enjoy quiet games	

5 Parameters achieved	Delayed development
7 "	Slightly delayed "
8 to 10 "	Satisfactory "

3–4 Years Development	Date of Notice
1. Puts on his shoes	
2. Counts 1 to 100	
3. Unbuttons own clothes	
4. Rides a tricycle	
5. Identifies basic colours	
6. Identifies different shapes	
7. Speaks short sentences	
8. Identifies A.B.C.D.	
9. They remember rhymes	
10. Repeats a simple story	

5 Parameters achieved	Delayed development
7 "	Slightly delayed "
8 to 10 "	Satisfactory "

Any special point noted ______________________